# Peak Performance Through Nutrition and Exercise

050823-N-3443B-001 Coronado, Calif. (Aug. 23, 2005)? Basic Underwater Demolition/Sea, Air and Land (SEAL) students take part in? Log PT.? Teammates work through their second hour of log physical training at the Naval Special Warfare Center in Coronado. Navy SEALs are named after the environment in which they operate, the Sea, Air, and Land, and are the foundation of Naval Special Warfare combat forces. U.S. Navy photo by Robert Benson (RELEASED)

# Peak Performance Through Nutrition and Exercise

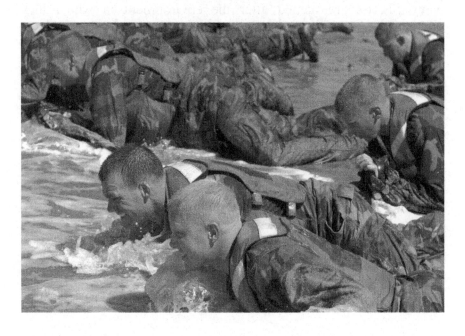

Anita Singh, Ph.D., RD, Tamara L. Bennett, M.S.
and Patricia A. Deuster, Ph.D., M.P.H.

Department of Military and Emergency Medicine
Uniformed Services University of the Health Sciences
F. Edward Hebert School of Medicine

080820-N-2959L-328 CORONADO, Calif. (Aug. 20, 2008) Basic crewman training (BCT) students crawl through the surf during their final training evolution at Naval Amphibious Base, Coronado. The final training evolution, known as the "Tour," is a three-day, two-night training session in which the students are tested physically and mentally on what they have learned during the seven-week program. BCT is the first phase of special warfare combatant-craft crewman (SWCC) training. SWCCs operate and maintain the Navy's inventory of state-of-the-art, high performance boats used to support SEALs in special operations missions worldwide. (U.S. Navy photo by Mass Communication Specialist 2nd Class Dominique M. Lasco/ Released)

# Foreword

Funding to develop this guide was received from Health Affairs, Department of Defense (DoD). Our project was one of many health promotion and prevention initiatives selected for funding. The selection of this project indicated a need for resources and materials that address the health and fitness needs of military personnel. We recognize that there are numerous books, tapes and websites dedicated to physical fitness and performance nutrition for the general public. However, our goal was to develop a comprehensive resource that is specifically tailored to address the unique physical fitness and nutrition requirements of Navy personnel. Our previous publications include "*The Navy SEAL Nutrition Guide*" and "*The Navy SEAL Physical Fitness Guide*". We hope that the nutrition and fitness information in this guide will help you achieve both your professional physical readiness and your personal performance goals. A companion guide for use by health promotion personnel is entitled "*Force Health Protection: Nutrition and Exercise Resource Manual.*"

# Acknowledgments

We would like to acknowledge the following for reviewing the book entitled "Force Health Protection: Nutrition and Exercise Resource Manual" on which this guide is based:
From Bureau of Medicine (BUMED):

CAPT Janee Przybyl
From Bureau of Naval Personnel (BUPERS):

LCDR Sue Hite and LCDR Neil Carlson
From Navy Environmental Health Center (NEHC):

Ms. Mary Kay Solera, Ms. Sally Vickers and Ms. Diana Settles
From Navy Supply Systems Command (NAVSUP):

CDR Al Siewertsen, Ms. Pam Beward and Ms. Andrea Andrasi
From the Uniformed Services University of the Health Sciences (USUHS):

COL Jeannette E. South-Paul

Our thanks go to the following individuals whose photographs appear in this guide: HM2 Jeanette Miller, HN Ellen Tate, HM1 (FMF) Rico Renteria, HM1 (SW/AW) Michael Mitchell, HM2 (FMF) Keith Avery, J02 Cerise Fenton, Dr. Jeffrey Bennett, and Dawn Schultz. Also, many thanks to HM1 (FMF) Otis B. Brown, the USUHS Brigade, and Morale, Welfare, and Recreation (MWR) for allowing us to take pictures during the Navy PRTs and the MWR sponsored events. We also want to acknowledge Mr. Gene Jillson from Defense Visual Information Center for providing us with the Navy images that appear throughout this guide.

Disclaimer: The opinions and assertions expressed herein are those of the authors and should not be construed as reflecting those of the Department of the Navy, the Uniformed Services University of the Health Sciences (USUHS), or the Department of Defense.

# Introduction

As documented in enclosure (1) of OPNAV6110.1E, it is the responsibility of each service member to:

♦ Maintain a lifestyle that promotes optimal health and physical readiness.

♦ Develop a regular, year-round, fitness program of aerobic, flexibility, and muscular strength and endurance exercises using resource information and the assistance of the Command Fitness Coordinator (CFC) and recreational services departments.

This guide has been prepared to assist you in your efforts to gain or maintain a high level of physical fitness by combining sound nutritional and physical fitness practices. An overview of basic nutrition and physical fitness programs including aerobic conditioning and strength training are provided. Information for designing exercise programs for individuals at various levels of physical fitness is provided in this guide. Because deployment is part of a Navy career, the importance of nutrition and exercise in maintaining physical readiness when deployed is discussed in Chapters 10 and 12. Also, many people take nutritional supplements to enhance physical performance. The benefits and risks associated with using performance enhancing supplements is discussed in Chapter 14. In another chapter (Chapter 15) women's issues such as nutrition and exercise during pregnancy and lactation are discussed. Moreover, resources used to prepare this guide, including websites for various Naval Commands and Civilian organizations involved in health promotions, are provided in Appendix D.

Seek the assistance of health promotion staff in your command. They have the knowledge and experience to help you attain your health and fitness goals. We encourage you to use this guide and hope that the ideas presented in Chapter 17 (Adopting Healthy Habits) will enable you to form healthy eating practices and to exercise regularly.

Anita Singh, Ph.D., RD, LN
Tamara L. Bennett, M.S., ACSM certified Health and Fitness Instructor
Patricia A. Deuster, Ph.D., M.P.H., LN

Department of Military and Emergency Medicine
Uniformed Services University of the Health Sciences
F. Edward Hebert School of Medicine

# Table of Contents

10

# List of Figures

# List of Tables

# List of Worksheets

# 1 | Energy Balance and Body Composition

In this chapter you will learn about:

♦ Energy balance.

♦ Estimating energy needs.

♦ Body composition and body fat distribution.

Maintaining a healthy body weight and body fat percentage through sound dietary and exercise practices helps to ensure optimal health, fitness, and physical performance. All of these issues are relevant in maintaining military readiness and force health protection, and in promoting optimal health of military personnel. This chapter introduces you to the basic concepts of energy balance and body composition.

## Energy Balance

Energy balance is the difference between the number of kilocalories (kcals or Calories) you eat (intake) and the number of kcals you burn (output).

### Figure 1-1. Energy Balance: Intake vs. Output

Intake = Output,
i.e., energy balance.

Intake = 3000 kcal    Output = 3000 kcal   Weight Maintained

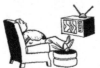 

Intake > Output,
i.e., positive energy
balance.

Intake = 4000 kcal    Output = 2000 kcal    Weight Gain

Intake < Output,
i.e., negative energy
balance.

Intake = 2000 kcal    Output = 3000 kcal    Weight Loss

Figure taken from FI Katch and WD McArdle. *Nutrition, Weight Control, and Exercise*, 3rd Ed. Philadelphia: Lea & Febiger, 1988.

14

# Sensitivity of Energy Balance

Energy balance can be changed by altering energy intake, energy output, or both, as shown in the following examples. (1 pound (lbs.) of fat equals 3,500 kcal.)

Example 1:
Eating 1 extra chocolate chip cookie (65 kcal) each day for 1 year would be: 65 kcal x 365=23,725 kcal. This would add up at the end of the year to a total net weight gain of 6.8 lbs. (23,725 ÷ 3,500).

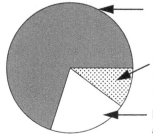

Example 2:
If you maintain your kcal intake and run an extra mile per day, 5 days per week, you would expend an extra 100 kcal/mile x 5 miles/week x 52 weeks = 26,000 kcals per year. This would result in a net weight loss of 7.4 lbs. per year (26,000 ÷ 3,500).

# Estimating Energy Needs

Energy needs are based on daily energy output or expenditures. The three major contributors to energy expenditure are:

### Worksheet 1-1. Calculate Your BMR

**Basal Metabolic Rate (BMR):** This is the energy needed to maintain life. Calculate your BMR using Worksheet 1-1.

**Digestion:** A small amount of energy is needed to digest food. This is accounted for in the BMR equation in Worksheet 1-1.

**Physical Activity:** Energy is needed during physical activity. Estimate your activity factor from Table 1-1.

15

## Table 1-1. Estimate Your Activity Factor

| | Level of Activity | Activity Factor |
|---|---|---|
| Very Light | Seated and standing activities, driving, playing cards, computer work. | 1.2 |
| Light | Walking, sailing, bowling, light stretching, golf, woodworking, playing pool. | 1.4 |
| Moderate | Jogging, aerobic dance, light swimming, biking, calisthenics, carrying a load. | 1.6 |
| Strenuous | Stairmaster, ski machine, racquet sports, running, soccer, basketball, obstacle course, digging, carrying a load uphill, rowing. | 1.9 |
| Exceptional | Running or swimming races, cycling uphill, hard rowing, carrying heavy loads. | 2.3 |

Your Activity Factor is _____.

## Total Daily Estimated Energy Requirement

Your total daily estimated energy requirement (EER) is the amount of kcals you need to eat each day to offset the energy expended through your BMR and physical activity and maintain an energy balance of zero. Calculate your EER in Worksheet 1-2.

**Worksheet 1-2. Calculate Your Estimated Energy Requirement (EER)**

Energy Needs = _____ X _____
          *BMR     *Activity Factor

Your Estimated Energy Requirement (EER) = _____kcal/day.

* Your BMR is calculated in Worksheet 1-1. The Activity Factor is from Table 1-1. The estimated energy needs of typical 19-50 year old men and women who are light to moderately physically active are 2,900 and 2,200 kcals/day, respectively.

By meeting your EER, you should have an energy balance of "zero" and maintain your current body weight. If your goal is to either lose or gain weight, adjust your kcal intake only slightly and engage in a well-rounded exercise program. A healthy goal when losing or gaining weight is to lose or gain 1/2 - 1 lbs. per week.

For specific questions about weight management and kcal requirements, consult the **Navy Nutrition and Weight Control Self-Study Guide** (NAVPERS 15602A at http://wwwnehc.med.navy.mil and http://www.bupers.navy.mil/services under "Navy Nutrition and Weight Control), or talk to a Registered Dietitian, your Command Fitness Coordinator, or your doctor. Also, see Chapter 3 to learn about eating healthfully.

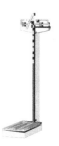

# Body Composition

The Body Mass Index (BMI) can be easily calculated to assess your body composition. Calculate your BMI in Worksheet 1-3 and compare it to the classifications.

### Worksheet 1-3. Calculate Your BMI

Your BMI = _____ x 705 ÷ (_____)$^2$ = _____.
body weight (lbs)                height (inches)                ratio

| Ratio: | Classification: |
|--------|-----------------|
| <20 | Underweight |
| 20-25 | Normal |
| 25-30 | Overweight |
| >30 | Obese |

The BMI classifications have been developed to identify individuals at risk for being either over- or underweight. However, BMI can misclassify some large frame or muscular people as overweight. It is strictly a ratio and does not necessarily reflect percent body fat accurately. If you feel your BMI incorrectly categorizes you, have your percent body fat measured by a trained professional. Body fat can be determined from a variety of techniques including hydrostati (underwater) weighing, skinfold measurements, and circumference measurements (as done in the Navy).

# Fat Distribution

In addition to BMI, it is helpful to know your waist-to-hip ratio (WHR). This ratio determines your pattern of fat distribution, i.e., where you store body fat. The formula for calculating waist-to-hip ratio is:

## Worksheet 1-4. Calculate Your Waist-to-Hip Ratio

Your WHR = _____ ÷ _____ = _____
             waist circumference (inches)   hip circumference (inches)       ratio

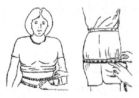

**Standards for Waist-to-Hip Ratios**

| Men: | <0.95 |
|------|-------|
| Women: | <0.80 |

Ratios greater than those listed above indicate a tendency toward central (torso) obesity. People who store excess fat in their mid-sections are at increased risk for heart disease and diabetes.

In the following chapters you will learn sound nutritional practices and ways to enhance your physical performance. Importantly, you will see how good nutrition and a balanced exercise program together influence your physical fitness, military readiness, and ultimately your overall health.

# 2 | Overview of Nutrition

In this chapter you will learn about:

♦ The different nutrients and their functions in the body.

♦ The various food sources of all the nutrients.

♦ Importance and distribution of water in the body.

There are six classes of nutrients: carbohydrates (CHO), proteins, fats, vitamins, minerals and water. CHO, proteins, and fats are energy providing nutrients, while vitamins and minerals are needed for energy metabolism. Water is the most abundant nutrient in the body and is essential for the normal functioning of all the organs in the body. All six nutrients will be discussed in detail throughout the chapter.

## Energy Providing Nutrients

The ideal percentage of daily kcals from CHO, proteins and fats for optimum health and performance are shown in the chart to the right.

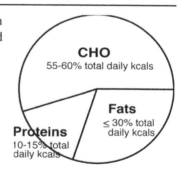

## Carbohydrates

CHO are found in grains, fruits, and vegetables and are the main source of energy in a healthy diet. CHO provide energy to the body in the form of glucose (stored as glycogen), act as building blocks for chemicals made by the body, and are used to repair tissue damage.

Unfortunately, many people think CHO are unhealthy and lead to weight gain. That notion came about because many people add high-fat toppings and sauces to their starchy foods.

The two types of CHO are:

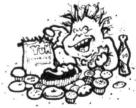

♦ **Simple CHO** - have one or two sugar molecules hooked together. Examples include: glucose, table sugar, sugars in fruits, honey, sugar in milk (lactose), maple syrup, and molasses. Simple sugars are added to some processed foods and provide extra kcals.

♦ **Complex CHO** - have three or more simple sugars hooked together and are digested into simple sugars by the body. Examples include: whole grains, fruits, vegetables, and legumes (peas, beans). Both **starch** (digestible) and **dietary fiber** (indigestible) are forms of complex CHO. Although, dietary fiber does not provide any kcals, for health reasons it is recommended that adults eat 20-35 grams of fiber a day. This is achieved by eating more fruits, vegetables, and whole grains.

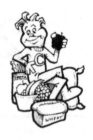

## Energy From CHO

 1 gram of CHO supplies 4 kcal.

CHO should supply 55-60% of your total daily kcals.

e.g., in a 2,000 kcal diet at least 2,000 x 55 ÷ 100 = 1,100 kcals should be from CHO. To convert kcals of CHO into grams of CHO, divide the number of kcals by 4; i.e., 1,100 kcals ÷ 4 kcals per gram = 275 grams of CHO.

### Worksheet 2-1. Calculate Your CHO Requirements

_____ x 0.55 = _____ kcal from CHO per day.
Your EER (from Worksheet 1-2)

_____ ÷ 4 kcal per gram =_____ grams CHO per day.
kcal from CHO per day

# Proteins

Proteins are found in meat, fish, poultry, dairy foods, beans and grains. Proteins are used by the body to form muscle, hair, nails, and skin, to provide energy, to repair injuries, to carry nutrients throughout the body, and to contract muscle.

## Energy from Proteins

Your protein needs are determined by your age, body weight, and activity level. Most people eat 100 to 200 g of proteins each day, which is more protein than is actually needed by the body. Many people eat high-protein foods because they think that proteins make them grow "bigger and stronger". Actually, these excess kcals from proteins can be converted to fat and stored. High-protein intakes also increase fluid needs and may be dehydrating if fluid needs are not met (see "Water" on Chapter 12).

### Table 2-1. Determining Your Protein Factor

**Grams of Proteins Per Pound of Body Weight**

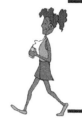

| Activity Level | Protein Factor |
|---|---|
| Low to Moderate | 0.5 grams |
| Endurance Training | 0.6 - 0.8 grams |
| Strength Training | 0.6 - 0.8 grams |

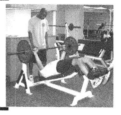

Your Protein Factor is _____.

Calculate your daily protein requirements in Worksheet 2-2 using your protein factor from Table 2-1.

### Worksheet 2-2. Calculate Your Protein Requirements

_____ X _____ = _____ grams of proteins per day.
Body Weight (lbs.)    Protein Factor

# Fats

Fats are an essential part of your diet, regardless of their bad reputation. Fats provide a major form of stored energy, insulate the body and protect the organs, carry nutrients throughout the body, satisfy hunger, and add taste to foods. However, not all fats are created equal. The three types of fats naturally present in foods are saturated, and mono- and polyunsaturated fats. A fourth type of fat, trans fat, is formed during food processing.

- ♦ **Saturated Fats** are solid at room temperature and are found primarily in animal foods (red meats, lard, butter, poultry with skin, and whole milk dairy products); tropical oils such as palm, palm kernel and coconut are also high in saturated fat.

- ♦ **Monounsaturated Fats** are liquid at room temperature and are found in olive oil, canola oil and peanuts.

- ♦ **Polyunsaturated Fats** are liquid at room temperature and are found in fish, corn, wheat, nuts, seeds, and vegetable oils.

Saturated, monounsaturated, and polyunsaturated fats should each be less than or equal to 10% of your total daily kcals. Therefore, total fat intake should be less than or equal to **30%** of your total daily kcal intake.

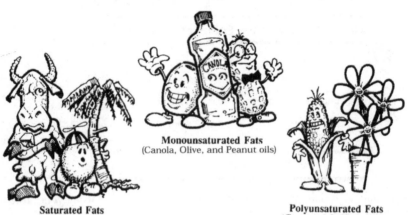

**Monounsaturated Fats**
(Canola, Olive, and Peanut oils)

**Saturated Fats**
(Animal fats and tropical oils)

**Polyunsaturated Fats**
(Corn and Safflower oils)

♦ **Trans Fats** are created when foods are manufactured. Currently, food labels do not list the trans fat content of a food but if "hydrogenated oils" are listed under ingredients it indicates the presence of trans fats. The more processed foods you eat, the greater your trans fat intake. Trans fats may increase blood cholesterol.

A high-fat diet is associated with many diseases, including heart disease, cancer, obesity, and diabetes. On average, people who eat high-fat diets have more body fat than people who eat high-CHO, low-fat diets. On the other hand, a fat-free diet is also very harmful since fat is an essential nutrient.

## Energy From Fat

> 1 gram of fat supplies 9 kcal, more than twice the energy supplied by CHO.
>
> Fats should supply no more than 30% of your total daily kcals.

e.g., in a 2,000 kcal diet no more than 2,000 x 30 ÷ 100 = 600 kcals should be from fats. To convert kcals of fat into grams of fat, divide the number of kcals by 9; i.e., 600 kcals ÷ 9 kcals per gram = 67 grams of fat.

### Worksheet 2-3. Determine Your Maximum Fat Limit

_____ x 0.30 = _____kcal of fat per day.
Your EER(from Worksheet 1-2)

_____ ÷ 9 kcal per gram =_____grams of fat per day.
kcal of fat per day

# Cholesterol

Cholesterol is made in the liver, is an essential part of body cells, serves as a building block for some hormones (e.g., testosterone and estrogen), and it is required to digest fats. Cholesterol is also consumed in the diet by eating animal products. High intakes of dietary cholesterol and saturated fats are associated with an increased risk for heart disease. The American Heart Association recommends that daily cholesterol intakes should not exceed 300 milligrams (mg.). Red meats and egg yolks are examples of cholesterol rich foods that should be consumed in moderation.

# Vitamins and Minerals

Vitamins and minerals do not provide kcals but both facilitate release of energy from CHO, proteins, and fats. Specific functions of each are listed in Table 2-2 and Table 2-3.

## Vitamins

Vitamins are classified as fat or water soluble.

◆ **Fat Soluble Vitamins** are absorbed with dietary fat and can be stored in the body. These include vitamins A, D, E and K.

◆ **Water Soluble Vitamins** are not stored in the body and excess is excreted in the urine. These include the B and C vitamins.

## Minerals

Minerals are classified according to their concentrations and functions in the body.

◆ **Minerals** - examples include: calcium and magnesium.

◆ **Trace Minerals** - are less abundant than minerals; examples include: zinc, copper and iron.

◆ **Electrolytes** - examples include sodium, potassium and chloride.

## Recommended Dietary Allowances

The Recommended Dietary Allowances (RDA) and the Dietary Reference Intakes (DRI), shown in Table 2-2 and Table 2-3, are the amounts of the vitamins and minerals that a healthy person should eat to meet the daily requirements. Your vitamin and mineral needs can be met by eating a variety of foods. However, if you elect to take vitamin and mineral supplements, you are urged to take only the RDA/DRI amount for each micronutrient (see Chapter 14,). Taking more than the RDA of a micronutrient could lead to toxicity and create deficiencies of other micronutrients.

## Vitamins and Minerals in the Diet

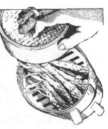

No one food has all of the vitamins and minerals, so you need to eat a variety of foods. Food preparation, medications, caffeine, tobacco, alcohol, and stress can all affect the amount of nutrient available to the body. For example, drinking coffee or tea with meals can decrease iron absorption and taking antibiotics can increase your Vitamin B needs.

Some cooking tips to minimize vitamin and mineral losses include:

♦ Use just enough water to prevent burning.

♦ Cook vegetables only until they are crisp and tender.

♦ Steam or stir-fry foods to retain the most vitamins.

♦ Cut and cook vegetables shortly before serving or store them in an airtight container.

 The nutrient content of many foods can be found on food labels. Also, you can look up information for most foods on the US Department of Agriculture's (USDA) web site (http://www.nal.usda.gov/fnic/foodcomp/data) or consult a dietitian or nutritionist.

# Table 2-2. Requirements and Functions of Vitamins

| Fat Soluble Vitamins | Some Important Functions | Food Sources |
|---|---|---|
| **Vitamin A:**<br>Retinol, Retinoids, Carotene<br>800-1,000 $\mu$g. RE or 5,000<br>International Units (IU). | Growth and repair of body tissues, immune function, night vision. Carotene is the water soluble form with antioxidant properties. | Oatmeal, green and yellow fruits and vegetables, liver, milk. |
| **Vitamin D:**<br>5-10 $\mu$g. or 200 - 400 IU. | Regulates calcium metabolism and bone mineralization. | Fortified milk, egg yolk, salmon, sunlight. |
| **Vitamin E:**<br>alpha-Tocopherol, 8-10 mg. | Antioxidant, protects cell membranes, and enhances immune function. | Fortified cereals, nuts, wheat germ, shrimp, green vegetables. |
| **Vitamin K:**<br>60 - 80 $\mu$g. | Assists in blood clotting and calcium metabolism. | Green and leafy vegetables. |
| **Water Soluble Vitamins** | **Some Important Functions** | **Food Sources** |
| **Vitamin $B_1$:**<br>Thiamin, 1.0 -1.5 mg. | Needed in energy metabolism, and growth. Supports muscle, nerve, and cardiovascular function. | Fortified cereals, legumes, pork, nuts, organ meats, molasses, yeast. |
| **Vitamin $B_2$:**<br>Riboflavin, 1.2 -1.7 mg. | Essential for energy metabolism; growth and tissue repair. | Cereals, liver, milk, green leafy vegetables, nuts, whole grains. |
| **Vitamin $B_3$:** Niacin,<br>Niacinamide, Nicotinic acid<br>13 -19 mg. | Essential for energy metabolism and nerve function. | Lean meat, seafood, milk, yeast, enriched cereals, whole grains. |
| **Vitamin $B_5$:**<br>Pantothenic acid, 4 - 7 mg. | Essential for energy metabolism and for nerve function. | Legumes, meat, fish, poultry, wheat germ, whole grains. |
| **Vitamin $B_6$:**<br>Pyridoxine HCl, 2 mg. | Essential for CHO and protein metabolism, immune function, red blood cell production, nerve function. | Oatmeal and cereals, banana, plantain, poultry, liver. |
| **Folate:**<br>Folic acid, Folacin, 400 $\mu$g. | Vital for red blood cell synthesis. Essential for the proper division of cells. Maternal folate deficiency may result in an infant with birth defects. | Fortified cereals, green leafy vegetables, liver, lentils, black-eyed peas, orange juice. |
| **Vitamin $B_{12}$:**<br>Cobalamin, 2 $\mu$g. | Required for red blood cell production, energy metabolism, and nerve function. | Ground beef, liver, seafood, milk, cheese. |
| **Biotin:**<br>30 - 100 $\mu$g. | Participates in energy metabolism, fatty acid formation, and utilization of the B vitamins. | Legumes, whole grains, eggs, organ meats. |
| **Vitamin C:**<br>Ascorbic acid, Ascorbate<br>60 mg. | Antioxidant, role in growth and repair of tissues, increases resistance to infection, and supports optimal immune function. | Cantaloupe, citrus fruit, strawberries, asparagus, cabbage, tomatoes, broccoli. |

From the 1989 RDA and 1998 DRIs for healthy adults 19 to 50 years. CHO = carbohydrates. mg= milligrams, $\mu$g= micrograms.

## Table 2-3. Requirements and Functions of Minerals

| Mineral | Some Important Functions | Food Sources |
|---|---|---|
| Boron<br>Unknown | Important in bone retention. | Fruits, leafy vegetables, nuts, legumes, beans. |
| Calcium<br>1,000 - 1,300 mg. | Essential for growth and structural integrity of bones and teeth; nerve conduction; muscle contraction and relaxation. | Yogurt, milk, cheese, tofu, fortified juices, green leafy vegetables. |
| Chromium[1]<br>50 - 200 $\mu$g. | Participates in CHO and fat metabolism; muscle function; increases effectiveness of insulin. | Whole grains, cheese, yeast. |
| Copper[1]<br>1.5 - 3 mg. | Essential for red blood cell production, pigmentation, and bone health. | Nuts, liver, lobster, cereals, legumes, dried fruit. |
| Iron[2]<br>10 -15 mg. | Essential for the production of hemoglobin in red blood cells and myoglobin in skeletal muscle, and enzymes that participate in metabolism. | Liver, clams, oatmeal, farina, fortified cereals, soybeans, apricot, green leafy vegetables. |
| Magnesium<br>280 - 350 mg. | Essential for nerve impulse conduction; muscle contraction and relaxation; enzyme activation. | Whole grains, artichoke, beans, green leafy vegetables, fish, nuts, fruit. |
| Manganese[1]<br>2 - 5 mg. | Essential for formation and integrity of connective tissue and bone, sex hormone production, and cell function. | Nuts, legumes, whole grains. |
| Phosphorous<br>800 - 1,200 mg. | Essential for metabolism and bone development. Involved in most biochemical reactions in the body. | Fish, milk, meats, poultry, legumes, nuts. |
| Potassium[3]<br>2,000 mg. | Essential for nerve impulse conduction, fluid balance, and for normal heart function. | Squash, potatoes, beans, fresh fruits (bananas, oranges) and vegetables (tomatoes). |
| Selenium<br>55 - 70 $\mu$g. | Antioxidant, works with vitamin E to reduce oxidation damage to tissues. | Meats, seafood, cereals. |
| Sodium[4]<br>500 - 2,400 mg. | Essential for nerve impulse conduction, muscle contraction, fluid balance, and acid-base balance. | Table salt, canned and processed foods. |
| Zinc<br>12 - 15 mg. | Involved in metabolism, immune function, wound healing, and taste and smell sensitivity. | Seafood, beef, lamb, liver, eggs, whole grains, legumes, peanuts. |

From the 1989 RDA and 1998 DRIs for healthy adults 19 to 50 years. CHO = carbohydrates. [1]Estimated safe and adequate daily intake range - meets requirements of individuals and avoids the danger of toxicity (Food and Nutrition Board, 1989). [2]Men should consult a physician before taking iron supplements. [3]The minimum daily requirement for potassium is 2,000 mg. [4]The minimum daily requirement for sodium is 500 mg. or 1,250 mg. of salt. Salt is 40% sodium and 60% chloride. One teaspoon of salt (5g sodium chloride) has 2g (2,000 mg) of sodium. mg= milligrams, $\mu$g= micrograms.

# Water

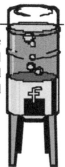

Approximately 60% of total body weight is water. Thus, adequate amounts of water must be consumed daily to ensure the normal functioning of the body and to replenish lost fluids. Water is needed to help digest and absorb nutrients, excrete wastes, maintain blood circulation, and maintain body temperature

**Worksheet 2-4. Calculate Your Daily Water Requirement**

Your Body Weight = _____lbs.

0.5 x _____(body weight) ÷ 8 oz. per cup = _____ cups per day.

Note: Exercise, heat, cold, and altitude can increase fluid requirements. See Chapters 11 and 12.

## Maintaining Fluid Balance

Fluid balance, like energy balance, is determined by the ratio of fluid losses to fluid intakes. With dehydration, water loss exceeds intake and fluid balance becomes negative. Water is lost in the urine, in stools, in sweat, and through breathing. When activity levels are low, most fluids are lost through the urine. When activity levels are high or the temperature is high, most of the fluid is lost through sweat. To maintain fluid balance you must consume enough fluids each day.

## Dehydration

Dehydration results when fluid losses exceed fluid intake. Conditions that can lead to dehydration include:

♦ Not drinking enough fluids daily.

♦ Working or exercising in a hot environment (wet or dry).

♦ Working or exercising in a cold environment (wet or dry).

♦ Going to high altitudes.

♦ Drinking too much alcohol or exercising with a hangover.

If 4% of your body weight is lost through fluid losses, decision-making, concentration, and physical work are impaired. A loss of 20% of body water can result in death (see Figure 2-1).

27

## Figure 2-1. Symptoms of Dehydration

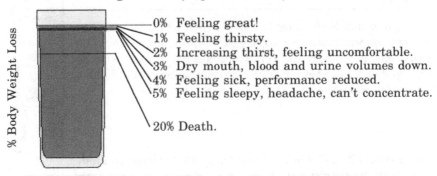

% Body Weight Loss

- 0% Feeling great!
- 1% Feeling thirsty.
- 2% Increasing thirst, feeling uncomfortable.
- 3% Dry mouth, blood and urine volumes down.
- 4% Feeling sick, performance reduced.
- 5% Feeling sleepy, headache, can't concentrate.

20% Death.

## Worksheet 2-5. Calculate Your Water Loss Limit

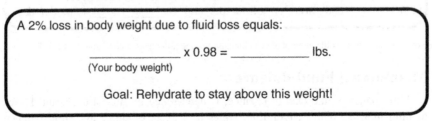

A 2% loss in body weight due to fluid loss equals:

_____ x 0.98 = _____ lbs.
(Your body weight)

Goal: Rehydrate to stay above this weight!

Chapter 3 outlines the dietary guidelines which apply the information discussed throughout this chapter to everyday dietary practices and food choices.

# 3 | Eating for Optimal Health and Fitness

In this chapter you will learn about:

♦ Dietary Guidelines.

♦ The Food Guide Pyramid.

♦ Food labels.

♦ Nutrient-dense foods.

♦ Vegetarian diets.

♦ Eating out wisely.

You have heard the saying "You are what you eat". That is because what you eat makes a difference in how you perform, how you feel, and affects your long-term health. This chapter provides information on how to follow healthy dietary practices whether you are eating at home, in a galley, or at a restaurant.

## Dietary Guidelines for Americans

The US Department of Agriculture (USDA) and the Department of Health and Human Services (DHHS) prepared Dietary Guidelines for all Americans 2 years of age and older. (http:\\www.nal.usda.gov/fnic/dga). The seven guidelines are:

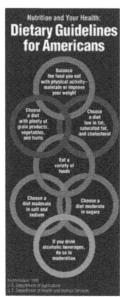

1. Eat a variety of foods.

2. Balance the food you eat with physical activity - maintain or improve your weight.

3. Choose a diet with plenty of grain products, vegetables, and fruits.

4. Choose a diet low in fat, saturated fat and cholesterol.

5. Choose a diet moderate in sugars.

6. Choose a diet moderate in salt and sodium.

7. If you drink alcoholic beverages, do so in moderation.

For more specific guidance on food selection, the USDA and the DHHS developed the food guide pyramid in Figure 3-1.

# The Food Guide Pyramid

You must have noticed the food guide pyramid on food labels. The USDA and the DHHS designed this pyramid to be a flexible dietary guide for Americans. Each compartment contains a different food group and the recommended number of servings that should be consumed daily. The primary energy-providing nutrient (Chapter 2) found in each food group is written in parenthesis. See Figure 3-1.

## Figure 3-1. Food Guide Pyramid

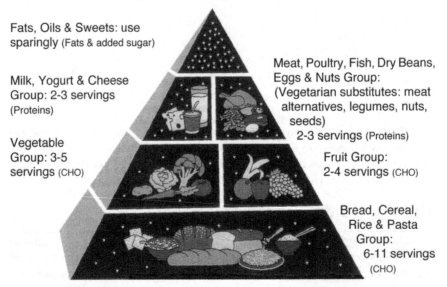

Fats, Oils & Sweets: use sparingly (Fats & added sugar)

Milk, Yogurt & Cheese Group: 2-3 servings (Proteins)

Vegetable Group: 3-5 servings (CHO)

Meat, Poultry, Fish, Dry Beans, Eggs & Nuts Group: (Vegetarian substitutes: meat alternatives, legumes, nuts, seeds) 2-3 servings (Proteins)

Fruit Group: 2-4 servings (CHO)

Bread, Cereal, Rice & Pasta Group: 6-11 servings (CHO)

Although this Food Guide Pyramid is found on most food labels, many people are unsure how to use its information. The most common questions are about serving sizes and how many servings should be eaten. Often people overestimate the size of a serving, thereby eating more kcals than they anticipated. Table 3-1 gives an estimate of the amount of food per serving for each food group and Table 3-2 lists the number of servings required from each food group to meet the various total daily kcals shown in the left column. Look up the number of servings you need from each of the food groups to meet your Estimated Energy Requirements (EER, Worksheet 1-2).

## Table 3-1. Portion Sizes Equivalent to a Serving

| Food Group | Serving Size |
|---|---|
| Bread, Cereal, Rice, Pasta & Grains | 1 slice of bread, 1/2 cup cooked rice or pasta, 1 oz.* breakfast cereal, 1/2 bagel. |
| Vegetables | 1 cup leafy vegetables, 1/2 cup raw or cooked vegetable, 3/4 cup vegetable juice. |
| Fruits | 1 medium size fruit, 1/2 cup canned fruit, 3/4 cup of 100% fruit juice, 1/4 cup dried fruit. |
| Milk, Yogurt, & Cheese | 1 cup milk or yogurt, 2 oz. cheese. |
| Meat, Poultry, Fish, Dry Beans, Eggs, Nuts | 3 oz. lean meat, poultry, fish, 1 egg, 2 Tbsp* peanut butter, 1/2 cup cooked beans. |
| Fats, Oils, Sweets | 1 tsp* oil, 1 pat of butter, 1 Tbsp salad dressing or sour cream. |

*oz. = ounces, Tbsp. = tablespoon, tsp = teaspoon.

## Table 3-2. Suggested Servings Based on Total Daily Caloric Intake

| Total Daily Kcals | NUMBER OF SERVINGS PER FOOD GROUP | | | | | |
|---|---|---|---|---|---|---|
| | Bread | Vegetables | Fruits | Meats | Milk | Fat grams |
| 1,400 | 6 | 4 | 3 | 2 | 2 | <47 |
| 1,600 | 7 | 5 | 4 | 2 | 2 | ≤53 |
| 1,800 | 8 | 5 | 4 | 2 | 3 | ≤60 |
| 2,000 | 10 | 5 | 4 | 2 | 3 | ≤67 |
| 2,200 | 11 | 5 | 4 | 3 | 3 | ≤73 |
| 2,400 | 12 | 6 | 5 | 3 | 3 | ≤80 |
| 3,000 | 15 | 6 | 6 | 3 | 3 | ≤100 |

Adapted from Navy Nutrition and Weight Control Self-Study Guide, NAVPERS 15602A 1996, p. 44.

# 5-A-Day

You may have heard of the national campaign to increase the amount of fruits and vegetables eaten by all Americans. This campaign, called "5-a-Day" has been adopted by all military services. Its purpose is to encourage people to eat at least five servings of fruits and vegetables each day. Following this program can add needed vitamins and minerals to your daily food

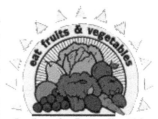

5 a Day–for Better Health!

31

intake; cut your risk of heart disease, cancer and digestive diseases; help control cholesterol; prevent constipation; and can help manage your body weight and percent body fat. Additionally, many fruits and vegetables contain "antioxidants" (see Glossary) and other nutrients that can be beneficial to your health. Some ideas to incorporate more fruits and vegetables in your diet can be found in Appendix A.

# Food Labels

To fully understand and use the information in the Food Guide Pyramid you need to understand how to read nutrition labels on foods. An example of a food label is shown in Figure 3-2.

**Figure 3-2. How to Read a Food Label**

Serving size reflects the typical amount of the food that many people eat.

The list of nutrients displays the amount in one serving of the food.

Ingredients are listed from the most to the least abundant items found in the food.

**Nutrition Facts**

Serving Size 8 fl oz (240 ml)
Servings Per Container 8

**Amount Per Serving**

**Calories** 100   Calories from Fat 20

% Daily Value*

| | |
|---|---|
| **Total Fat** 2.5g | 4% |
| Saturated Fat 1.5g | 8% |
| **Cholesterol** 10mg | 3% |
| **Sodium** 130mg | 5% |
| **Total Carbohydrate** 12g | 4% |
| Dietary Fiber 0g | 0% |
| Sugars 11g | |
| **Protein** 8g | |

| | | |
|---|---|---|
| Vitamin A 10% | • | Vitamin C 4% |
| Calcium 30% | • | Iron 0% |
| Vitamin D 25% | | |

* Percent Daily Values are based on a 2,000 calorie diet. Your daily values may be higher or lower depending on your calorie needs:

| | | Calories | 2,000 | 2,500 |
|---|---|---|---|---|
| Total Fat | | Less than | 65g | 80g |
| Sat Fat | | Less than | 20g | 25g |
| Cholesterol | | Less than | 300mg | 300mg |
| Sodium | | Less than | 2,400mg | 2,400mg |
| Total Carbohydrate | | | 300g | 375g |
| Dietary Fiber | | | 25g | 30g |

Ingredients: Lowfat milk, Vitamin A palmitate, Vitamin D₃

The % Daily Values are based on a 2,000 kcal diet. Use the number to compare the amount of nutrients found in various foods.

Percentage of the daily vitamin and mineral recommendation that is met in one serving of the food.

# Selecting Nutrient-Dense Foods

Foods that contain the most nutrients in the fewest kcals are called **nutrient-dense foods**. Now that you know the number of kcals and importance of all the nutrients, can you select foods that provide many nutrients without consuming too many kcals? Let us equate this concept to bargain shopping. If you have $10 and you need to buy several toiletries, you will buy the products that cost the least money yet still meet your needs. The same should be true with respect to the amount of kcals in the foods you eat. For example, compare the nutritional content of skim milk and whole milk.

| | Skim Milk | Whole Milk |
|---|---|---|
| **Total kcal** | **85** | **157** |
| grams CHO | 12 | 11 |
| grams proteins | 8 | 8 |
| **grams fat** | **0** | **9** |
| mg Calcium | 303 | 290 |

Skim milk and whole milk contain the same amounts of proteins, CHO, and calcium; however, skim milk has less total kcals and less fat than the whole milk. Therefore, you can drink two glasses of skim milk for the same amount of kcals as 1 glass of whole milk, yet you will get twice the proteins, CHO, and calcium.

The goal of selecting nutrient-dense foods is not to avoid fat grams, but rather to select foods that contain the essential nutrients without eating an overabundance of kcals.

# Vegetarian Diets

The popularity of vegetarian diets has increased in recent years. One reason is that vegetarian diets have been linked to lower risks for several diseases, including heart disease, high blood pressure, and diabetes. There are many different types of vegetarian diets. The similarities among them lie in their emphasis on grains, vegetables, fruits, beans, and nuts to obtain all the necessary nutrients. The main concern people have when deciding to try a vegetarian diet is whether the diets will meet their vitamin, mineral, and protein needs. These needs can be met if vegetarians include foods from all the food groups in the pyramid. Meat, fish and poultry can be substituted with legumes, nuts, seeds, and other meat alternatives. Strict vegetarians who omit animal products from their diets may need to take Vitamin $B_{12}$ and calcium supplements.

# Eating Out

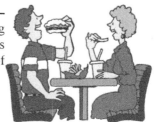

On many occasions you may find yourself eating away from home. Following the dietary guidelines when dining out is a very important aspect of optimizing your health, fitness, and performance.

## Tips for Eating Out

♦ Order foods high in complex CHO (see Chapter 2,).

♦ Choose foods that are baked, broiled, steamed, poached, smoked, roasted, grilled, flame-cooked, or marinara.

*On average, Americans eat 1 of 3 meals away from home each day.*

- Order sauces and dressings "on the side."
- Trim all visible fat off the meat.
- Order a salad as your appetizer.
- Order dessert after you have eaten your main course and only if you are still hungry.
- Limit alcohol consumption.
- Avoid foods that are fried, breaded, battered, flaky, crispy, creamy, au gratin, puffed, loaded, or tempura. Also, avoid hollandaise and bearnaise sauces.
- Many restaurants have a listing of the nutritional content of their foods available on request, even fast food restaurants. More information can be found at the USDA's web site at: http:\\www.nal.usda.gov/fnic.

# Snacking

Many people think snacking is unhealthy and leads to weight gain because many people don't eat healthy snacks! If you enjoy snacking and you want to maintain your body weight and perform well, then selecting healthy snacks is critical. Think through a typical day. How often and where do you usually snack? Are your snacks healthy or loaded with extra kcals? Follow these tips to help promote healthy snacking! (Snacks should not replace a meal.)

- Choose foods such as fruits, vegetables, plain popcorn, dried fruits, whole grain crackers, pretzels, cereal snack mixes, unsweetened fruit juices, fresh produce, and low-fat yogurt.
- Snack on fresh fruits or vegetables with low-fat peanut butter or low-fat cheese spreads.
- If you must have candy, choose one that is high in CHO and as low in fat as possible.

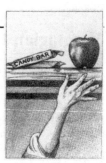

Many people replace high-fat snacks with the low-fat alternatives in an attempt to lower their total fat intake. Be cautious, however, because even low-fat snacks can lead to weight gain and increases in body fat when too many kcals are consumed. Remember: low-fat does not mean low in kcals, so do not over eat!

# Nutrition
# Throughout Life

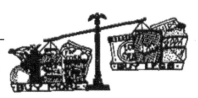

The guidelines discussed in this chapter can be applied to everyone throughout their lifetime. Identify when your energy needs are changing (i.e., changes in physical activity levels, pregnancy, breast feeding) and adjust your diet appropriately to maintain your health and fitness. Each individual should eat the appropriate number of servings from each food group based on their EER (refer to Chapter 1 and Table 3-2). Seek the help of a Registered Dietitian if you have any concerns about your diet or the diet of a family member. Even if you do not cook your meals or if you eat in the galley, you can make healthy food choices (see Appendix A). When eating in the galley, ask for the **Healthy Navy Options** menu items (available in the larger galleys and ships). Make high-fat foods the exception rather than the rule in your diet.

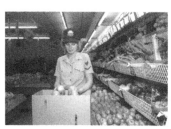
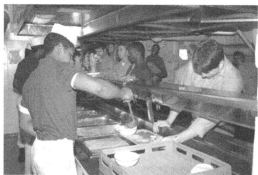

# 4 | Overview of Physical Fitness

In this chapter you will learn:

 ♦ The definition of physical fitness.

 ♦ The benefits of being physically fit and its relation to military readiness.

 ♦ The FITT Principle.

 ♦ The Physical Fitness Pyramid.

 ♦ Fuel used during exercise.

 ♦ Exercise Sequence.

 ♦ Training and Detraining.

In the military, physical fitness is emphasized because of its role in military readiness and force health protection. Many jobs in the Navy require personnel to handle heavy equipment, to adapt quickly to harsh environments, and to work in limited quarters. Training for these situations ensures that you are physically able to perform these tasks repeatedly, without fail, whenever the need arises. In short, this is the rationale for optimizing your physical fitness levels and for performing PRT tests every six months! (See OPNAV6110.1E at http://www.bupers.navy.mil/ services under "New Navy PRT Program" for the PRT standards).

> "Fitness, which has been defined as the matching of an individual to his physical and social environment, has two basic goals: health and performance [which lie on a continuum]. Physical fitness requirements in the military consist of a basic level of overall fitness required for health of all individuals and a higher level of fitness that is required for the performance of occupational activities...In addition to this, the military must address the need for ongoing, job-specific performance training."
> IOM (1998) Physical Fitness Policies and Programs, in Assessing Readiness in Military Women, p. 64.

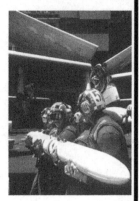

# What is Physical Fitness?

What does it mean to be physically fit? The American College of Sports Medicine (ACSM) has defined physical fitness as a set of characteristics (i.e., the work capacity of your heart and lungs, the strength and endurance of your muscles, and the flexibility of your joints) that relate to your ability to perform physical activities. Regular physical activity leads to improved physical fitness and many other physiologic, cosmetic, and psychological benefits. Depending on personal goals 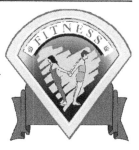 and job requirements the level of physical fitness to attain can range from basic, health-related to more specific, performance-related fitness (Figure 4-1).

## Figure 4-1. The Fitness Continuum

| **Health-related** | **General** | **Performance-related** |
|---|---|---|
|  | 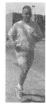 |  |
| Lowers stress, increases metabolism, promotes health, prevents disease. | Increases muscle and heart and lung fitness, leads to a healthy body composition, improves flexibility. Most Navy personnel are in this category. | Enhances specific physical tasks or skills. For Navy personnel who perform physically demanding tasks. Also, for people competing in organized sports. |

# FITT Principle

There are four basic components in all physical fitness programs. These are frequency of exercise, intensity of the exercise, time spent exercising, and the type of activity. These are outlined in the Physical Activity Pyramid in Figure 4-2 and are called the **FITT Principle** guidelines.

### FITT = Frequency, Intensity, Time & Type

## The Physical Activity Pyramid

Just as the nutrition guidelines are outlined in the Food Guide Pyramid (Chapter 3), the guidelines for physical activity are diagrammed in the Physical Activity Pyramid (Figure 4-2). This pyramid was designed to help people live an active lifestyle, reap the fitness and performance benefits of routine exercise, reduce the health risks associated with inactivity, and reduce the injury risks associated with too much activity.

# Figure 4-2. The Physical Activity Pyramid

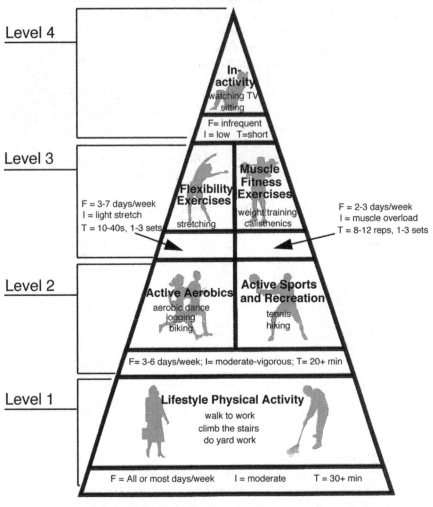

Level 4

In-activity
watching TV
sitting
F= infrequent
I = low    T=short

Level 3

Flexibility
Exercises
F = 3-7 days/week
I = light stretch
T = 10-40s, 1-3 sets      stretching

Muscle
Fitness
Exercises
weight training
calisthenics

F = 2-3 days/week
I = muscle overload
T = 8-12 reps, 1-3 sets

Level 2

Active Aerobics
aerobic dance
jogging
biking

Active Sports
and Recreation
tennis
hiking

F= 3-6 days/week; I= moderate-vigorous; T= 20+ min

Level 1

Lifestyle Physical Activity
walk to work
climb the stairs
do yard work

F = All or most days/week      I = moderate      T = 30+ min

F = frequency; I = intensity; T = time; exercise Type is in bold

Adapted from CB Corbin and RP Pangrazi. Physical Activity Pyramid Rebuffs Peak
Experience. *ACSM's Health and Fitness Journal* 1998; 2(1): pages 12-17.

The four levels are arranged according to their FITT principle recommendations.
Activities at the base of the pyramid should be performed more frequently than the
activities found at the top of the pyramid. Level 1 activities include household
chores, walking to work, and walking up and down stairs. Level 2 activities include
aerobic exercises and participation in sports and recreational activities. Level 3
consists of strength and flexibility exercises, while Level 4 includes sedentary
activities, such as watching TV. Do Level 1-3 activities each day to get the most
health benefits.

# Fuel Used During Exercise

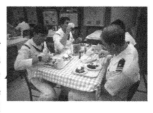

Before discussing the various exercise guidelines in the following chapters, here is an overview of how your body makes fuel for exercise. Your body uses the CHO, fats, and proteins you eat to make a chemical called **adenosine triphosphate (ATP)**. You need ATP to contract your muscles during exercise. ATP can be made two ways. The first makes ATP without using oxygen and is called the **anaerobic energy system.** The second requires oxygen to make ATP and is called the **aerobic energy system**. Both of these systems are required during most activities but, depending on the duration and intensity of the activity, there is a greater reliance on one system over the other. Exercises lasting less than 5 minutes rely most on the anaerobic energy system, while exercises lasting more than 5 minutes rely most on the aerobic energy system.

# Exercise Sequence

An exercise sequence to follow to improve exercise performance and reduce the risk of injury is outlined in Figure 4-3. Note that it includes warming-up, stretching, and cooling-down.

**Figure 4-3. Recommended Exercise Sequence**

1. Warm-Up

↓

2. Stretch (Dynamic)

↓

3. Physical Activity Session*

↓

4. Cool-Down

↓

5. Stretch (Static)**

*Refer to the exercises found in Levels 2 and 3 of the Physical Activity Pyramid.
**For more information on stretching see Chapter 9.

- A **warm-up** gradually increases muscle temperature, metabolism, and blood flow to prepare you for exercise and lengthen short, tight muscles. Warm-up for at least 5 minutes before exercise.

- A **cool-down** is important because it may help reduce muscle soreness after your workout. Cool-down for at least 5 minutes by exercising at a light pace using the same muscles just exercised.

- **Rest** is an exceedingly important factor in recovery from strenuous workouts. Hard workout days should be followed by easy workout days or rest to give your body time to fully recover.

## Training and Detraining

Training and detraining are responsible for gains and losses, respectively, in fitness levels. Training according to the FITT Principle guidelines will lead to optimal fitness benefits. On the other hand, decreases in fitness due to detraining occur at twice the rate of training gains when physical activity stops completely (Table 4-1).

### Table 4-1. Training vs. Detraining

| Training | Fitness Component | Detraining |
|:---:|:---:|:---:|
| ↑ | Heart and lung function | ↓ |
| ↓ | Resting heart rates | ↑ |
| ↑ | Muscle strength and endurance | ↓ |
| ↑ | Resting metabolism | ↓ |
| ↑ | Muscle fuel (glycogen) stores | ↓ |
| ↑ | Ability to sweat and dissipate body heat | ↓ |

Detraining can be minimized by maintaining your usual exercise intensity, even if the frequency and duration of workouts is decreased. This concept is important for you to understand, as you may have limited time and fitness equipment available while deployed for extended periods. Ironically, it is in these situations that you depend most on your physical fitness to perform your duties. Therefore, learn the basic training principles and how to work around equipment, space, and time limitations (see Chapter 10).

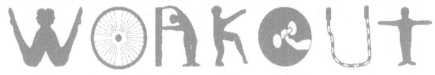

# 5 | Cardiorespiratory

# Training

In this chapter you will learn about:

- ♦ The physiology of the heart and lungs.
- ♦ Benefits of cardiorespiratory training.
- ♦ The FITT Principle guidelines for cardiorespiratory training.
- ♦ Aerobic-training program design and progression.

Cardiorespiratory activities make up the bulk of the physical activities in Levels 1 and 2 of the Physical Activity Pyramid (Chapter 4, Figure 4-2). These activities improve health and fitness by increasing the work capacity of the heart and lungs. Other terms used to describe these activities include

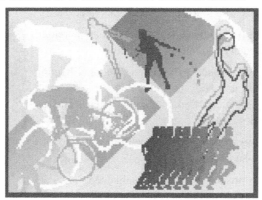

## Cardiorespiratory Physiology

The heart is a muscle that is required to contract continuously throughout your life to deliver oxygen to all organs in the body. Your lungs breathe in oxygen and breathe out carbon dioxide. Blood vessels connect the heart and lungs so that carbon dioxide can be removed from the blood and oxygen can be added to the blood. The heart then pumps this blood throughout the body. During exercise your heart must pump more often and more strongly to supply oxygen to your exercising muscles to make energy. In turn, you breathe in more often and more deeply to increase the amount of oxygen you inhale and carbon dioxide that you exhale.

41

The basis of cardiorespiratory training is to place greater demands on the heart (e.g., make the heart beat more times per minute) than what is required during rest. This results in a stronger heart that can pump more blood and deliver more oxygen to the body per heart beat, and a lower resting heart rate. Since most daily activities are aerobic in nature, improving the delivery of oxygen to the muscles will improve your work performance. (See "Fuel Used During Exercise" on page 26.) So, view your heart as an aerobic muscle that must be conditioned for optimum functional health and fitness throughout your life.

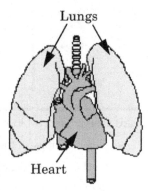
Lungs

Heart

# Benefits of Cardiorespiratory Exercise

The benefits of cardiorespiratory, or aerobic, conditioning include:

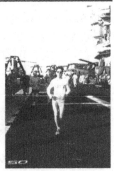

- ♦ A stronger heart and lower resting heart rate.
- ♦ Fitness and performance benefits, such as increased aerobic capacity and muscle endurance.
- ♦ Health benefits, such as maintenance of a healthy body weight and body fat percentage, management of stress, and decreased blood cholesterol and fat (triglycerides) levels.

- ♦ Increased performance in physically-demanding jobs such as lift-and-carries.
- ♦ Increased muscle tone and enhanced physical appearance.

# Aerobic Exercise Guidelines

The FITT Principle guidelines discussed in Chapter 4 and outlined in the Physical Activity Pyramid for cardiorespiratory training are:

- ♦ **Frequency** - 3-7 days per week.
- ♦ **Intensity** - 60% to 90% of maximum heart rate (Max HR).
- ♦ **Time** - 30-60 minutes per day within your target heart rate zone.
- ♦ **Type** - continuous, low resistance, high repetition activities.

The guidelines for exercise "intensity" and "type" are discussed next.

## Intensity of Exercise

Intensity can be estimated using the following measures:

## Target Heart Rate Zone

Measuring increases in heart rate during a workout is a quick and easy method to gauge the intensity of your workout. To measure your heart rate follow the instructions in Figure 5-1.

**Figure 5-1. Measuring Heart Rate at the Wrist**

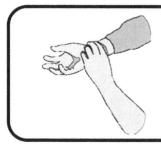

◆ Use your fingertips, not your thumb, to find your pulse at your wrist below your thumb.

◆ Count the beats for 10 seconds.

◆ Multiply this number by 6 to get your heart rate in beats per minute (bpm).

Once you measure your exercising heart rate how do you know whether you are exercising at the appropriate intensity? Depending on your age and fitness level there is a target heart rate zone that is appropriate for your exercise intensity. Use Figure 5-2 or Worksheet 5-1 to find your target heart rate zone.

See "Training Design and Progression" on page 33 to determine what heart rates, within this range, you should aim for during exercise based on your level of physical fitness and your fitness goals.

**Figure 5-2. Target Heart Rate Zones**

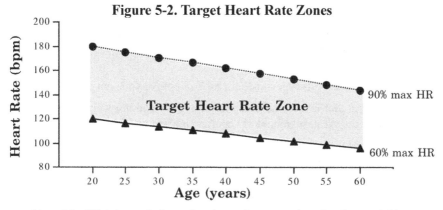

Note: Max HR is lower during swimming and arm exercises. For these activities, subtract 13 from Max HR before calculating your target training zone.

43

**Worksheet 5-1. Determine Your Target Heart Rate]**

Age-Predicted Max HR = 220 - _____ your age = _____ bpm.

60% max HR = _____ max HR x 0.60 = _____ bpm.

90% max HR = _____ max HR x 0.90 = _____ bpm.

Target HR Zone = _____ to _____ bpm.

## Calories

Most exercise machines display "Calories" during an exercise session and the term is very familiar to most people. Calories per hour is the amount of energy you use when maintaining the same exercise intensity for an hour.

## Perceived Exertion

Ratings of Perceived Exertion, or RPE, are the subjective measures of exercise intensity perceived by the exerciser. Measurements are based on a twenty-point scale, "6" is no exertion and "20" is maximal exertion. Most people should workout at a perceived exertion of 12 to 15 (moderate to hard).

## Other Measures of Exercise Intensity

**METs** and **Watts** are two other measures of exercise intensity that are often calculated on exercise machines. A MET (metabolic equivalent) describes the amount of energy needed to perform an activity. Rest requires 1 MET, so exercising at 5 METs requires 5 times the energy needed at rest. A Watt is the amount of work (kcal) performed in a given time period. Therefore, the greater the watts (kcal/min), the higher the exercise intensity.

## Type of Exercise

Continuous, low-resistance exercises (e.g., biking) train the heart and muscles to use oxygen more efficiently. To choose the best exercises for you to perform, consider the following:

♦ Training is exercise specific; e.g., run to improve your run time.

♦ Exercises that involve several muscle groups and are weight bearing will require the greatest amount of Calories to perform.

♦ Exercises that you enjoy the most are the best exercises for you.

♦ Alleviate boredom and decrease your risk for injuries by alternating the types of exercise you perform, i.e., **cross-train**.

## Table 5-1. Examples of Aerobic Exercise

| Activity | Advantages | Comments |
|---|---|---|
| Aerobic Classes | Group setting, variety of levels | Work at your own pace; ask instructor prior to class for any tips. |
| Bicycling | Low impact, good for cross-training | Bike at 70 rpms, with a slight bend in knee to best work the quadriceps muscles. |
| Climbing (Stairclimbing) | Weight bearing | Uses major muscles of lower body; weight-bearing (by not leaning arms on machine); Rock climbing strengthens upper body, too. |
| Cross-country Skiing | Low impact, good for cross-training | Uses most major muscle groups. |
| Jumping Rope | Can be performed in small quarters | A fast pace mimics running; wear good shoes and avoid cement surface. |
| Martial Arts | Group setting | Popular; many classes focus on flexibility, strength, and relaxation. |
| Rowing | Low impact | Works most major muscle groups. |
| Running | Minimal gear required | High impact, alternate with other exercises. |
| Swimming, water aerobics | No impact, can be a group setting | Uses most major muscle groups; great as a primary, cross-training, or rehab. exercise. |
| Walking | Low impact, minimal gear | Uses most major lower body muscle groups; weight-bearing. |

There are several variations to these basic types of exercises, such as kickboxing, treading, and spinning.

## Cross-Training

For overall health and general fitness benefits, and to avoid overuse injuries, alternate the types of exercises you perform, i.e., cross-train. Cross-training allows you to build a good aerobic base while avoiding overuse injuries caused by the repetitive motions of a single exercise. Engaging in a variety of activities (e.g., alternating between running and swimming) uses different muscle groups.

For performance-related fitness, strategies to enhance your speed for activities that require fast, short-duration sprints (like soccer) are presented in Table 5-2.

45

**Table 5-2. Various Training Strategies for Speed**

| Workout | Description |
|---|---|
| Intervals | Ratios of recovery to work; i.e., 3 minutes normal (recovery) pace, 1 minute sprint (work) pace (3:1); 30 second recovery to 15 second work (2:1), etc. |
| Fartleks (Speed Play) | Mix normal exercise pace with hard exercise pace in an unstructured pattern. |
| Time Trial | Exercise for predetermined distance at a race pace. |
| Pyramids | Exercise is divided in stages as follows: 1 minute (min) hard: 1 min rest, 3 min hard: 2 min rest, 5 min hard: 3 min rest, 7 min hard: 5 min rest, then work back down (5:3, 3:2, 1:1). |
| Sprint | Maximum exercise effort lasting 5-10 seconds, followed by complete recovery. |
| Acceleration Sprint | Jog 100 yards (yds.), then sprint 100 yds., then walk 100 yds.; repeat this pattern for a given distance or time. |

# Training Design and Progression

You want to tailor your program to realistically meet your goals and time demands, so answer the questions honestly (see Chapter 17 for more information on setting goals).

♦ If you have been sedentary, begin by increasing your physical activity by performing more daily activities, found in Level 1 of the Physical Activity Pyramid (Figure 4-2).

♦ Once you can easily perform these activities, add 5-10 minutes of Level 2 activities two to four days per week.

♦ Gradually increase the duration of the Level 2 activities by 10% per week until you can perform 20 to 60 minutes continuously. Your training intensity should be between 60% and 75% of your max HR (see Worksheet 5-1).

♦ Exercise at 80% to 90% of maxHR should only be performed by individuals in excellent physical fitness.

**The golden rules of training progression are:**

♦ Increase only one FITT component, i.e., frequency, intensity, time, or type, at a time.

♦ Increase your training by no more than 10% each week. Allow yourself time to adjust to this new routine before you increase your workout again. Increasing too fast will lead to injury and overtraining (see Chapter 13).

♦ Signs of overexertion include pain in your chest, breathlessness or gasping for breath, nausea, and dizziness. If you have any of these symptoms, stop exercising immediately!

Based on your answers to the questions above and your current fitness level, set up a weekly routine with moderate to hard workout days and rest days (Appendix B). You will add a strength training workout to this schedule in Chapter 7.

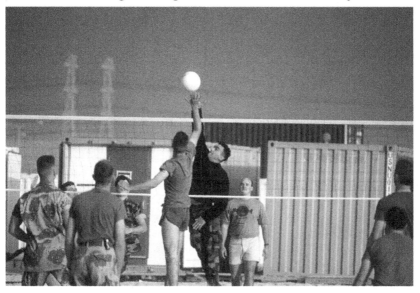

# 6 | Walk, Run, Swim!

In this chapter you will learn to:

♦ Design a walking program.

♦ Design a running program.

♦ Design a swimming program.

Walking, running, and swimming all provide excellent aerobic workouts. These three types of exercise will be discussed in this chapter for two reasons: 1) walking and running are the most common types of exercise that people engage in, and 2) all three modes of exercise can be used to test your level of physical fitness on the Navy PRT tests.

## Walking and Running Gear

To maintain or improve your fitness and avoid injuries while walking and running you need to use the right exercise gear. Below are some tips and information to help you purchase training gear.

♦ **Shoes** provide shock absorption, cushioning, motion control and durability. The proper shoes will help correct biomechanical problems, such as foot **pronation** (inward roll of your ankle) and arch height. Specialty stores, magazines, and web sites have a lot of information about the latest footwear and what footwear is best for your foot type. Do not buy shoes based on their brand name!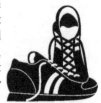

♦ **Orthotics** are shoe inserts that provide additional foot support and control for people with biomechanical conditions that may cause pain while running. They can be purchased as overthe-counter inserts or custom-made. Consult a sports medicine specialist or podiatrist.

♦ **Heart Rate Monitors** gauge exercise intensity by continuously monitoring heart rate. These consist of a wrist watch and a chest strap: the chest strap detects your heart beat and transmits it to the watch which displays heart rate in beats per minute. This allows you to check and maintain your heart rate within your target training zone (see Chapter 5) while you exercise.

♦ **Reflectors** and portable **beverage containers** are great for your safety and health when exercising outdoors. Other gear, such as walkmans, can provide entertainment, however, consider your training environment to determine whether they will hinder your safety by decreasing your awareness of your surroundings.

# Walking

Walking is the easiest, most common, low impact exercise that people engage in. However, there are many misconceptions about the usefulness of walking for weight loss and cardiorespiratory conditioning. These health benefits can be realized by walking, as long as the intensity is high enough to increase your heart rate to 60-75% of your max HR (Worksheet 5-1).

When you walk, keep your back straight and your stride comfortable. **Do not use ankle or hand weights** because they increase the stresses placed on your joints. If you have been sedentary, start by walking for 15 minutes on a flat surface at a pace that allows you to talk somewhat easily. Walk every other day. Each week increase the time you walk by 10% until you can walk for 20 minutes continuously. Next, increase your distance by 10% each week (staying at the 3.0 m.p.h. pace) until you can walk continuously for 2 miles. Then follow the program outlined in Table 6-1.

### Table 6-1. Outline of a Walking Program

| Weeks | Frequency times/week | Miles | Goal Time (min)/ pace | Comments |
|-------|------------|-------|----------------------|----------|
| 1-2 | 3 | 2.0 | 40 min / 3.0 m.p.h* | Quicken your pace by 1 min each week |
| 3-4 | 4 | 2.0 | 38 min / 3.2 m.p.h. | |
| 5-6 | 5 | 2.0 | 36 min / 3.3 m.p.h. | |
| 7 | 5 | 2.0 | 34 min/ 3.5 m.p.h. | Increase your distance by 1/2 mile each week |
| 8 | 5 | 2.5 | 43 min/ 3.5 m.p.h. | |
| 9 | 5 | 3.0 | 51 min/ 3.5 m.p.h. | |
| 10-15 | 5 | 3.0 | 45 min/ 4.0 m.p.h. | Maintain HR at 60% -75% of max HR. |
| 16-17 | 4 | 3.5 | 53 min/ 4.0 m.p.h. | |
| 18-19 | 4-5 | 4.0 | 60 min/ 4.0 m.p.h.** | |

Adapted from OPNAVINST 6110.1D Jan. 1990. *m.p.h. = miles per hour; ** add hills for variety.

# Running

A running program should only be started if you are able to walk 4 miles at a 4.0 m.p.h. pace. There are several reasons to begin a running program, such as managing your body weight, increasing your cardiovasclar fitness, and building your self-esteem.

## Running Form

Regardless of your running goals, pay attention to your form. This will ensure your running style is efficient and safe for your joints. The key is to run naturally and remain relaxed. Do not overstride, i.e., straightening your leg and landing with your heel in front of your knee. Overstriding is hard on the knees, back and the hips and can cause injuries.

**Figure 6-1. Three Traits of a Good Running Form**

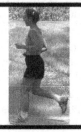

**Run Tall**

**Run Relaxed**

**Run Naturally**

## Running Surfaces

The best outdoor running surfaces are unbanked, smooth cinder tracks or artificially surfaced tracks. Concrete and asphalt sidewalks and roads are often banked and provide no shock absorption. Always change the direction you run on a track or path from one session to the next to reduce any biomechanical problems that may result from track conditions and repetition. Most treadmills are state of the art in terms of cushioning and you can control the speed and intensity of your workout. Deep water or aqua running is mainly used for rehabilitation as it takes the pressure off muscles and joints while providing cardiovascular benefits.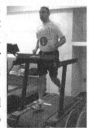

## Beginning a Running Program

When starting a running program, combine walking and jogging. Gradually increase the time spent jogging and decrease the time spent walking. Remember that your exercise intensity should be between 60%-75% of your max HR, so adjust your pace accordingly. Table 6-2 outlines a beginning jogging program to help make your transition easier. Advance to the next phase once you can consistently perform the walk-jog cycles outlined within your target heart rate zone. If you are

50

interested in running for fitness, a good goal is 6 to 8 miles per week, spread over 3 running days of 2 to 3 miles each. Start a running log to track your workouts (Worksheet B1), noting mileage, time, heart rate, and perceived exertion (see Chapter 5).

### Table 6-2. Beginning a Jogging Program

| Phases | Walk | Jog | Time / Distance | |
|--------|------|-----|-----------------|--|
| Phase 1: | 1 to 2 min. | Work up to jogging 2 min. continuously. | 20-30 min | |
| Phase 2: | 1 to 2 min. | Quarter mile (1 lap on a 440 meter track). | Jog six, quarter mile laps. | Check heart rate frequently. It should be between 60 and 75% max HR. (see Worksheet 5-1). |
| Phase 3: | 1 min. | Half mile (2 laps on a 440 meter track). | Jog three, half mile laps. | |
| Phase 4: | during warm-up and cool-down | 1 mile continuously. | 1-mile jog and 1-mile walk. | |
| Phase 5: | during warm-up and cool-down. | Increase jog by quarter-mile increments until running 2 to 3 miles continuously. | 2 to 3 miles. | |

## Increasing Your Running Workout

Once you can comfortably run 6-8 miles per week and you desire to progress further in a running program, start by increasing either your mileage or pace. Increasing either your distance or pace too quickly can cause training injuries, so gradually increase one at a time by no more than 10% per week. (i.e., if you can run five miles, increase your distance by a half mile and keep your pace constant.) Maintain this new distance for at least one week, or until it is consistently easy for you. Consistency is more important than speed. When running for exercise and not competition, your pace should be even (60-75% max HR) and allow you to talk comfortably.

### Increase your mileage or pace by only 10% per week.
### Do not increase your mileage and pace simultaneously.

Twenty to 30 miles per week is a good training distance for an intermediate runner (Table 6-3). As a rule, your risk of injury sharply increases as your running mileage increases. So, if running for fitness rather than competition, keep your weekly mileage below 30 miles. Beyond this, your injury risks far outweigh any additional fitness benefits. Cross-train to work on aerobic fitness without running more than 30 miles.

## Table 6-3. An Intermediate Running Program

| Week | Mon | Tues | Wed | Thur | Fri | Sat | Sun | Total |
|------|-----|------|-----|------|-----|-----|-----|-------|
| One | 2 | - | 2 | - | 2 | 2 | - | 8 |
| Three | 2 | - | 3 | - | 3 | 2 | - | 10 |
| Five | 3 | - | 3 | - | 3 | 3 | - | 12 |
| Seven | 3 | - | 4 | - | 4 | 3 | - | 14 |
| Nine | 3 | - | 4 | 3 | - | 3 | 4 | 17 |
| Eleven | 4 | - | 5 | 3 | - | 5 | 3 | 20 |
| Thirteen | 4 | - | 5 | 5 | - | 4 | 5 | 23 |
| Fifteen | 5 | - | 5 | 5 | - | 6 | 5 | 26 |
| Seventeen | 5 | - | 6 | 6 | - | 6 | 7 | 30 |

Miles

Cross train or rest on non-run days.

With an endurance base of 30 miles per week you can easily compete in 10Ks, the Army 10 Miler, and other similar events.

## Training for Long Distance Runs

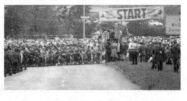

If you are interested in building an endurance base for running long distance races, such as a half marathon, the Marine Corps marathon, the Air Force Marathon, or similar events, contact a local running group, a national running program, or a trainer with experience in coaching distance runners. Training for these distance races can be very challenging, both physically and mentally. For more information on running distance races, contact the American Running and Fitness Association at http://americanrunning.org.

# Swimming

Swimming is an excellent exercise for overall fitness. Because the water supports your body weight, swimming is a great cross-training exercise for running and other high-impact activities. Swimming is also an alternative for people with orthopedic problems or those who are in rehabilitation.

## Beginning a Swim Program

For swimming to be your primary form of exercise, you must be a skilled swimmer. To emphasize the energy expenditure during a swim, swimming 1/4 mile, or 440 meters, is equivalent to jogging 1 mile. Therefore, it is very likely that an inexperienced swimmer will not be able to swim continuously for 20 to 30 minutes. If you are unfamiliar with the basic swimming strokes, focus on your technique by taking lessons. Once you swim continuously for 20-30 minutes you will have a good base for increasing your distance or pace. Table 6-4 outlines a 10-week swim program for intermediate swimmers.

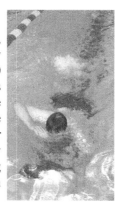

### Table 6-4. Swim Program to Build Your Distance

| Week | Distance (meters) | Number of Lengths | Frequency (Days/Week) | Goal Time (minutes) |
|------|-------------------|-------------------|-----------------------|---------------------|
| 1    | 300               | 12                | 4                     | 12                  |
| 2    | 300               | 12                | 4                     | 10                  |
| 3    | 400               | 16                | 4                     | 13                  |
| 4    | 400               | 16                | 4                     | 12                  |
| 5    | 500               | 20                | 4                     | 14                  |
| 6    | 500               | 20                | 4                     | 13                  |
| 7    | 600               | 24                | 4                     | 16                  |
| 8    | 700               | 28                | 4                     | 19                  |
| 9    | 800               | 32                | 4                     | 22                  |
| 10   | 900               | 36                | 4                     | 22.5                |

Table taken from OPNAVINST 6110.1D, Jan 1990, p 17.

## Open-Water Swimming

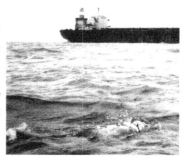

Open-water swimming can be a very challenging and rewarding workout. But before heading out to sea, you should be able to swim at least one mile continuously, and consistently, in a lap pool. When swimming in open water you are faced with many safety issues not addressed in pool training, so follow these safety rules: (Section adapted from L. Cox. *Seaworthy. Women's Sports and Fitness July-August* 1995;17(5):73-75.)

- sk lifeguards or locals about the safety of the area. (Are there any strong currents or riptides? What marine life is in the area? Avoid areas where sharks have been spotted.)

- Walk the beach along the course you will be swimming. Look at buoys, surfers, and other swimmers to gauge the direction and strength of the current. Pick landmarks (houses or lifeguard stations) to use as markers while you are swimming.

- Wear a comfortable, unrestricted suit (a wet suit in cold water); a swim cap and goggles with UVA/UVB protection. Water gloves and fins can be worn as well. Use a waterproof sunscreen all over your body.

- Never swim alone. On your first outing, swim just past the breaking waves.

- Follow the shoreline, staying 100 to 150 yards outside the breaking waves. Check your distance from the shoreline as you turn your head to breathe. Swim toward an unmoving target in the distance. Check your position with this target every 50 to 100 yards and adjust your course appropriately.

- A good starting distance for open-water swimming is a half mile. Swim against the current for the first quarter mile, then turn around and swim with the current for the last quarter mile. Gradually build up your distance by quarter mile increments.

- Avoid boats and jet skis by wearing bright colors. If a boat is moving toward you, swim away from it and kick hard to make large splashes that announce your presence.

# 7 | Strength Training

In this chapter you will learn about:

- ♦ Muscle strength.
- ♦ Muscle endurance.
- ♦ Strength training guidelines.
- ♦ Designing a strength training program.
- ♦ Proper training techniques.

Muscle strength and endurance training are essential components of overall fitness. Your ability to perform daily tasks and strenuous physical tasks can be enhanced by strength training. As you read through this chapter think about the physical tasks you perform routinely in your job or at home, the strength needed to perform those tasks, and which exercises mimic those tasks. The focus of your strength training routine should be functional or applied strength for job-specific activities, military readiness, and injury prevention. This chapter outlines the principles of muscle strength and muscle endurance training and the proper use of exercise equipment to help you achieve your goals.

## Strength versus Endurance

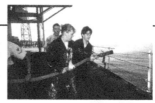

- ♦ Muscle strength is the force your muscle can exert against resistance. As you lift and lower a weight your muscle must generate enough force to move that weight.

- ♦ Muscle endurance is the ability of your muscle to repeatedly apply force to lift and lower a weight. Muscle endurance describes how long or how many times you can lift and lower a weight.

# Benefits of Strength Training

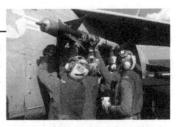

Strength training should complement aerobic workouts because each type of training results in different benefits. General benefits of strength training include:

♦ Increased muscle strength and muscle endurance, greater lean body mass, less body fat, and higher energy metabolism.

♦ Increased coordination and greater protection against injury.

♦ Increased self-esteem and less perceived stress.

♦ Better performance of physically-demanding, job-related tasks.

# Determinants of Muscle Size

Various factors influence muscle size (see Figure 7-1). Although some factors cannot be controlled, two factors that we can control are exercise and nutrition habits (Chapters 3, 4, and 11).

## Figure 7-1. Factors that Affect Muscle Size

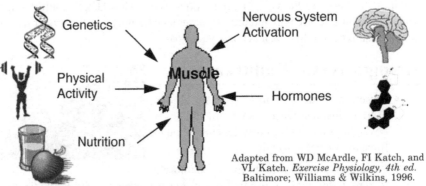

Adapted from WD McArdle, FI Katch, and VL Katch. *Exercise Physiology, 4th ed.* Baltimore; Williams & Wilkins, 1996.

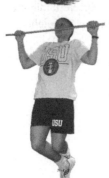

Men generally have more muscle mass than women, mainly because men produce more testosterone than women. Strength training may increase muscle mass slightly in women; however, a common **misconception** is that strength training will cause women to "bulk up." Importantly, strength training will greatly increase muscle strength and reduce the risks for injury. Moreover, women tend to have poor upper body strength and many military tasks require upper body strength.

# Strength Training Guidelines

## Training Form

Correct lifting techniques are critical for achieving maximum benefits and preventing injury (see Appendix C). If your form is incorrect, strength training can lead to injury, not strength gains.

+ Use minimal weight when learning a new exercise.

+ Use a closed grip (fingers and thumbs wrap around the bar or handle and touch each other), and place hands equidistant from the ends of the bar. Load the weights evenly across the bar.

+ For free weights, feet should be hip to shoulder width apart, knees slightly bent, and your back should keep its natural curve. Keep your head level and eyes focused straight ahead. If maintaining this posture is difficult than the weight is too heavy.

+ For resistance machines, adjust the pads to fit your body so the pads can support you during the lift. Keep your head level and eyes focused straight ahead.

+ **Lifts should be slow, smooth, and controlled.** Lift and lower the weight for 2-4 seconds in each direction to ensure that your muscle, not momentum, is moving the weight.

+ **Exhale** during the exertion (moving the weight against gravity), and **inhale** when returning to the start position. **Never hold your breath while exercising!**

+ Always use a spotter when lifting free weights.

The most common training errors occur when people focus on lifting the weight rather than focusing on stabilizing themselves and controlling the weight. The best way to avoid training mistakes is to ask a staff member at the gym to teach you new exercises and to suggest the best exercises for you based on your fitness level and goals. See Appendix C for examples of common errors in training techniques and how to avoid making them.

## FITT Principle Guidelines

Once you are comfortable with the basic training techniques for performing strength exercises, follow the FITT Principle, illustrated in the Physical Activity Pyramid (Chapter 4, Figure 4-2), to set up your routine. The FITT guidelines for strength training are:

+ **Frequency** - 2 to 3 times per week for each major muscle group on non-consecutive days.

+ **Intensity** - the total weight lifted or the resistance applied.

+ **Time** - the duration of the exercise.

+ **Type** - equipment used and the exercises performed.

Two terms you need to know are **repetition (rep)** and **set**. A rep is a single lifting and lowering of the weight. For example, one rep of a leg curl is lifting your ankle toward your buttocks, pausing one second, then returning your ankle to the start position. A set is the number of reps performed without stopping to rest. For example, if you perform 10 leg curls, rest for 60 seconds, followed by another 10 leg curls, you would have performed 2 sets, each of 10 leg curls. When recording the number of sets and reps performed, write **"sets x reps"** (i.e., 2x10 for the leg curl example).

## Intensity of Exercise

Focus on the intensity of your training only **after** you have perfected your lifting form. The basis of strength training is to gradually increase the amount of weight that you lift during training to ultimately increase the amount of force your muscles are capable of generating. This is called **progressively overloading** the muscle to achieve gains in strength without causing injury. The following intensity guidelines for general strength gains are for beginners, for people who are restarting their routines after a break, and for people learning new exercises.

♦ Once your form is perfected (page 44), gradually increase the weight you are lifting until you reach a weight that you can lift only 12 times with good form. Finding this 12-rep weight will be trial and error at first.

♦ Your 12-rep weight will increase as you gain strength, so increase the weight you are lifting appropriately (but no more than 10% each week).

♦ Start a training routine consisting of one to two sets of 12 reps for each major muscle group (defined in "Type of Exercise" on page 46).

A long-term strength routine of one to two sets of 12 reps is excellent for maintaining and increasing general strength. In addition, this type of routine only takes about 30 minutes to perform. Once you have developed a solid strength and endurance base (after about eight weeks) you may be interested in pursuing more specific training goals. In general, the following guidelines apply to the various types of strength training goals:

♦ Muscle endurance - two to three sets, 12-15 reps with a 15-rep weight; 30-60 seconds rest between sets.

♦ Muscle hypertrophy (increase in muscle mass) - three to six sets, eight to 12 reps with a 12-rep weight; 30-90 seconds rest between sets.

♦ Muscle strength - three to five sets, two to eight reps with an 8rep weight; at least 120 seconds rest between sets.

**Note: Do not perform maximal lifts when strength training.**

# Type of Exercise

For maximum benefit and to decrease the risk of injury, pay attention to:

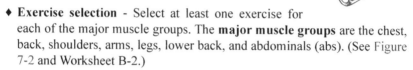

+ **Muscle balance** - perform exercises that target the opposing muscle groups across the joints to strengthen the major muscles and improve joint function; e.g., strengthen the biceps and triceps muscles in the upper arm.

+ **Exercise selection** - Select at least one exercise for each of the major muscle groups. The **major muscle groups** are the chest, back, shoulders, arms, legs, lower back, and abdominals (abs). (See Figure 7-2 and Worksheet B-2.)

+ **Exercise order** - perform multi-joint exercises before single-joint exercises. In a multi-joint exercise more than one joint (per side) moves during the exercise; e.g., your shoulders and elbows move during a bench press. In a single-joint exercise one joint (per side) moves during the exercise; e.g., only your elbow moves during an arm curl. Perform lower back and abdominal exercises at the end of your workout since those muscles are used for balance and posture during other exercises.

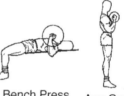

Bench Press     Arm Curl

Use Worksheet B-2 to design your workout and to record your training progress. Change the exercises you perform for each muscle group every four to eight weeks, even if you keep the same set and rep routine. Changing exercises will overload the muscles differently, increase your strength gains, and alleviate boredom. There are a variety of exercises for each muscle group listed in Figure 7-2. To increase their upper body strength, women should perform exercises that target the back, neck, chest, shoulders and arms.

## Figure 7-2. Exercises for Various Muscle Groups

**Neck**
(Trapezius)
shrug, pull-ups, rows

**Shoulder**
(Deltoid, Rotator Cuff)
lateral raise, upright row
shoulder press, bench press,
reverse fly, rotations

**Triceps**
triceps extensions, dip, push-up
bench presses, kickback

**Back**
(Latissimus Dorsi, Lats)
lat pulldown, pullover, rows
pull-up

**Low Back**
(Erector Spinae)
back extension, superman

**Forearm**
(wrist extensors)
reverse wrist curls

**Gluteals**
leg press, lunge, squats,
hip extension, glute-ham raise
rear thigh raise

**Hamstring**
leg curl, leg press, squats,
lunge, glute-ham raise

**Calf**
(Gastrocnemius & Soleus)
calf raise, heel raises, lunge

**Chest**
(Pectorals)
bench presses, chest fly, dip,
chest press, push-up

**Biceps**
curls (arm, preacher, hammer,
concentration), chin-up, rows
lat pulldown

**Abdominals**
(Rectus Abdominus and Obliques)
crunches, knee raises,
rotary torso

**Forearm**
(wrist flexors)
wrist curls

**Outer Thigh**
(hip abductors)
hip abduction, leg raises

**Quadriceps**
leg extension, leg press, squats, lunge, step ups

**Inner Thigh**
(hip adductors)
hip adduction, leg raises

**Shin**
(Tibialis Anterior)
toe raises, foot flexion with resistance

*BACK VIEW*          *SIDE VIEW*          *FRONT VIEW*

# Equipment

Strength training requires minimal personal gear: weights, a pair of supportive shoes, and lifting gloves. A weight lifting belt is only recommended during maximal or near maximal lifts, and is not recommended at all for exercises that do not stress the back. This is because the belt takes over the role of the abdominal muscles in stabilizing the torso, preventing the strengthening of the abdominal muscles.

The most common barbells found in gyms are Olympic style barbells. There are several styles that vary widely in size and weight, so ask a staff member at your gym to help you determine which barbell best suits your needs. In addition, the weight plates to load the barbells come in a variety of sizes and are measured in both pounds (lbs) and kilograms (kg). Pay attention to the weight measurements in your gym; there is a big difference between 10 lbs and 10 kg! Use adjustable collars to keep the plates on the bar.

Choosing which equipment to use depends largely on your goals and training experience. Table 7-1 lists a comparison of free weights and machines to help you with your choice. If you are new to a fitness center or if you are unsure how to work a piece of equipment, ask a fitness center staffer for an orientation. This orientation will help you design a workout routine based on the equipment selection at your gym.

Though this chapter focuses on resistance machines and free weights, resistance for strength training can come from a variety of sources. Other exercise techniques

60

and equipment available for strength training when space and equipment may be limited are outlined in Chapters 8 and 10.

### Table 7-1. Free Weights vs. Resistance Machines

| Free Weights | | Resistance Machines |
|---|---|---|
| Low cost and versatile. | | Expensive, less versatile, need access to equipment. |
| Form is crucial; spotter is needed. | 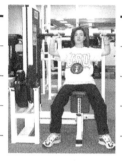 | Supports the body during the exercise; easy to adjust. |
| Trains balance and posture; mimics daily activities. | | Isolates muscle groups more easily than free weights. |
| Can perform multi-joint and single-joint exercises. | | Machines made for multi-joint and single-joint exercises. |
| Muscles trained through joint's full range of motion. | | Muscle training occurs in a limited range of motion. |

# Types of Workouts

The following two routines are basic workouts to build muscle strength. Choose the routine that is best for you based on the time available, your goals, your training experience, and your fitness level. More advanced workouts should only be performed once you have a solid muscle strength and endurance base and have perfected your lifting form. For more information on these more advanced routines (such as pyramids, super sets, and split routines) see your Command Fitness Coordinator or a certified fitness professional at your gym.

♦ **Full body workouts** -All the major muscle groups (as listed in Worksheet B-2) are exercised during a single session. Perform one to two sets of an exercise for each muscle group and rest between sets. This should take 20-45 minutes. For general strength training purposes; workout at least twice a week.

♦ **Circuit Training** - Combines aerobic and strength exercise stations. Each exercise station takes 30-45 seconds to perform and stations alternate between upper and lower body exercises. The circuit is repeated two or more times per session. Circuit training improves aerobic conditioning and moderately increases strength when performed three times per week. This routine is good for people who have less than 45 minutes to do both aerobic and strength exercises. (See Table 10-2 for an example.)

Use the guidelines in this chapter provided to develop a sound strength training program. Alternate exercises for each muscle group at least every eight weeks to maximize strength gains, enhance job-related fitness, and have fun!

# 8 | Calisthenics

In this chapter you will learn about:

♦ Proper form and guidelines for performing calisthenics.

♦ Designing a calisthenic exercise program.

♦ Abdominal exercise techniques.

Calisthenics require minimal equipment and can be performed in almost any location. These exercises can be used to develop and maintain muscle strength and muscle endurance, and can be particularly useful when strength training equipment is not available.

## Calisthenic Guidelines

When performing calisthenics to develop muscle strength or endurance, you should follow the same recommendations outlined in Chapter 7. Intensity is largely based on the number of sets and reps, and the length of rest periods. Resistance is provided by body weight rather than an external resistance. Proper form for calisthenic exercises follows many of the general exercise guidelines outlined in Chapter 7, including muscle balance and exercise order. Any of these exercises can be added to your gym-based routines to create more variety. Detailed instructions for some calisthenic exercises are in Table 8-1 (adapted from The Navy SEAL Physical Fitness Guide.)

To begin a calisthenics program select one exercise per muscle group from Table 8-1. Perform this routine two to three times per week.

♦ For each exercise, start with one set of eight reps. Rest 60 seconds after each set.

♦ Increase your workout each week by adding one to two reps until you can do 12 reps.

♦ Once you have reached this point, do two sets of eight reps of each exercise. Again, increase your workout by one to two reps per set each week until you can perform two sets of 12 reps.

♦ Once you have reached this point, do three sets of eight reps; again, increasing your workout by one or two reps per set each week until you can do three sets of 12 reps.

♦ Once you can do three sets of 12 reps, try increasing the difficulty of your workout by: 1) changing the exercises you perform; 2) decreasing your rest periods; 3) using a weighted pack or having a partner provide resistance; 4) exercising one side of the body at a time. Other suggestions are in Table 8-1.

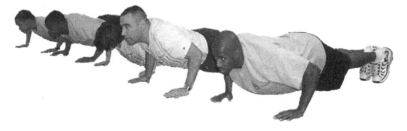

## Table 8-1. Calisthenic Exercises Arranged by Muscle Group

## NECK
**Neck Rotations**
Lie on back. Count 1: Lift head up and over to side. Count 2: Bring head to center; Count 3: Bring head to other side. Count 4: Return head to start position. Works neck flexors.

## LEGS

**Straight Leg Raise**
Sit on the edge of a bench, keeping back straight. Place hands behind you for support. Bend left knee 90o. Straighten right leg in front of you with your right heel resting on the deck. Count 1: Slowly raise your right leg, lifting it no higher than your hips, keeping your back straight. Count 2: Lower heel to 1 inch above the deck. Works hip flexors. Variation to increase difficulty: use an ankle weight.

**Hand to Knee Squat**
Place feet shoulder-width apart, arms at sides. Count 1: Bend at hip and knees, keep back straight and feet flat, until your fingertips pass knees. Knees should not go beyond toes. Count 2: Push through the heels to return to start position. Works quadriceps, hamstrings, and gluteals.

**Burt Reynolds**
Lie on left side with head supported by hand, bend right leg and place it in front of left knee. Count 1: Lift left leg 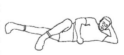 approximately 8 inches off deck. Count 2: Lower left leg to 1 inch above the deck. Repeat for the right leg. Works inner thigh (hip adductors

## Leg Lifts

Lie on left side, bend both knees at a 90o angle from torso. Count 1: Lift right leg 6-8 inches, keeping knee and ankle level. Count 2: Lower right leg to 1 inch above left leg. Repeat for the left leg. Works outer thigh (hip abductors).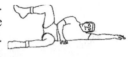

## One-Legged Squat

Shift weight to right leg, lifting the left leg straight out in front of you. Count 1: Bend right knee until it is over your toes. Count 2: Push up through right heel to return to start position. Repeat using other leg. Works quadriceps, hamstring, and gluteal muscles.

## Calf Raises

Stand on step with heels hanging off edge. Count 1: Lift heels 3 inches. Count 2: Lower heels 3 inches. Works calf muscles. Variations: Perform exercise with toes pointed inward, straight forward, and turned outward.

# GLUTEALS

## Rear Thigh Raises

Start on and knees and forearms. Lift left leg, keeping it bent 90o, so that left knee is no higher than hips. Keep back flat and hips level. Count 1: Lower left leg 6 inches. Count 2: Lift leg to start position. Switch legs and repeat. Works gluteals. Variation to increase difficulty: Straighten leg to be lifted.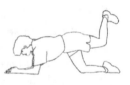

# LOWER BACK

## Superman

Lie on stomach. Count 1: Lift opposite arm and leg (i.e., right arm, left leg) 6 inches off deck. Hold for 3-5 seconds. Avoid hyperextension of the back. Count 2: Slowly lower arm and leg to deck. Repeat using opposite arm and leg. Works lower back and gluteals. Variation to increase difficulty: Add weights to arms and legs.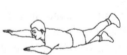

## Prone Back Extension

Lie face down, hands clasped behind back. Count 1: Lift upper torso until shoulders and upper chest are off Deck. Hold 3-5 seconds. Avoid hyperextension of back. Count 2: Return to start position. Works lower back. Variations to increase difficulty: Place hands behind back (easiest), behind head, straight over head (most difficult)

# CHEST, SHOULDERS, ARMS

## Push-Ups

Lie on stomach, feet together and hands shoulder width apart on deck, head facing forward, body straight. Extend arms. Count 1: Bend elbows 90o, lowering chest toward deck. Count 2: Return to start position. Works triceps, chest, shoulder, and abdominals.  **Variations:** Fingertip Push-ups - Begin as above, except use fingertips to support weight. Works forearms and improves grip strength. Triceps Push-ups - Begin as above, except place your  hands close together beneath your chest and spread fingers apart. Your thumbs and index fingers of both hands should almost touch.

## Dips

Rest hands on parallel bars. Extend arms; legs are not to support your weight unless needed for assistance. Count 1: Bend the elbows until 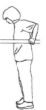 shoulders are level with the elbows. Count 2: Extend arms to return to start position. Works triceps, chest and shoulders.

# BACK, ARMS

## Pull-Ups

Begin from a dead hang on a horizontal bar, arms   shoulder-width apart, palms facing out. Count 1: Pull body up until chin touches bar. Do not kick. Count 2: Return to start position. Works the back and forearms. Grip variations: Narrow, Wide.

## Incline Pull-Ups

Using a low bar, lie or sit on the deck with chest under bar, 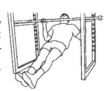 place hands shoulder-width apart on bar, palms out. Count 1: Pull upper body toward bar at a 45o angle. Squeeze shoulder blades together during movement. Count 2: Extend arms. Works back, shoulders, and arms.

## Chin-Ups

Begin from a dead hang (i.e., full extension) on a horizontal bar, arms  shoulder-width apart, palms facing in. Count 1: Pull body upward until chin touches top of bar. Do not kick. Count 2: Return to start position. Works the back, biceps.

# ABDOMINALS

## Crunches

Lie on back, knees bent 45o, hands behind head, elbows 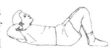 back. Count 1: Lift upper torso until shoulder blades are off the deck, tilt pelvis so lower back is pressed to the deck. Lead with the chest, not the head. Count 2: Return to start position. Works abdominals and obliques. Variations to increase difficulty: bring knees toward chest; extend legs vertically in the air; place a rolled towel under lower back. Arms may be placed (easy to most difficult) by sides, across chest, hands behind head, or hands clasped above head.

## Curl-up

Lie on back with knees bent, feet flat on deck, heels 10 inches from buttocks and anchored down. Cross arms and hands on chest or shoulders. Count 1: Curl torso up, touching elbows to upper thighs while hands remain on the chest or shoulders. Exhale as you lift. Count 2: Lie back until the lower edge of your shoulder blades touch the deck. Inhale as you lower. Works abdominals, obliques, and hip flexors. Note: Curl-ups are part of the Navy PRT. However, if you experience any lower back pain when performing curl-ups, try performing crunches instead.

OPNAVIST 6110.1E

---

# 9 | Flexibility

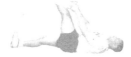

In this chapter you will learn about:

♦ The benefits of flexibility training.

♦ Physiology of stretching.

♦ Proper stretching techniques.

Flexibility training is an important component of a physical fitness program. If optimum functional fitness and military readiness are the goals, then well-balanced flexibility training is a must.

## Benefits of Stretching

Flexibility is the ability to move your joints freely through a full range of motion. The goal of flexibility training is to enhance joint movement while maintaining joint stability. Proper stretching increases flexibility, complements both strength and aerobic exercises, and leads to:

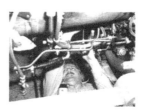

♦ Reduced muscle soreness after exercise.

♦ Lower risk for injury.

♦ Mental and physical preparation for exercise or competition.

♦ Enhanced muscle performance through a larger, functional range of motion.

♦ Mental relaxation.

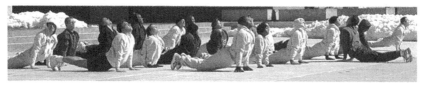

## Flexibility Exercises

One of the safest and most beneficial types of flexibility exercises is static stretching. **Static Stretches** are slow, controlled movements through a full range of motion. The term "static" means the stretch is held at the end of the joint's range of motion. These static exercises are considered safe and effective because they stretch the muscles and connective tissue without using fast movements that will be resisted by the muscles. These exercises can be done actively (e.g., you contract

67

the opposing muscle group to stretch the target muscle group) or passively (e.g., you use a towel to stretch the muscle). Incorporate the static stretches in Table 9-1 in your exercise program. These exercises target the muscle groups shown in Chapter 7, Figure 7-2. Select at least one stretch for each muscle group. Hold each stretch for 10-30 seconds then rest 10 seconds. Repeat each stretch 2-5 times. Muscle balance also applies to stretching, so stretch opposing muscle groups (e.g., stretch hamstrings and quadriceps). **Remember: static stretches should be performed slowly and held for 10 - 30 seconds.**

A second type of flexibility exercises is dynamic stretching (Table 9-2). **Dynamic Stretches** are controlled muscle contractions through a joint's range of motion. These stretches should be used to enhance the performance of an activity that immediately follows the stretch; i.e., swinging your racket prior to a tennis match. This type of stretching warms the muscles. Dynamic exercises are safe as long as you do not use momentum to force a joint through a greater range of motion than it is capable. Also, avoid bouncing movements.

## Table 9-1. Static Stretches

### Calf Stretch

Standing on a step, place the ball of the right foot on the edge of the step. Bend left knee and gently drop right heel. Stretches the right gastrocnemius. Variation: To stretch the ankle, slightly bend the right knee after dropping your right heel. Switch legs and repeat.

### Quadriceps Stretch

Lie on stomach with both legs extended. Slowly bend left knee. Gently grasp left ankle with right hand and pull toward body. Keep back straight. Stretches the quadriceps. Switch legs and repeat. Variation: Perform stretch when standing, holding on to a stationary object to keep your balance.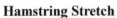

### Hamstring Stretch

Lie on back with both legs extended. Bring left leg to chest and grasp left thigh with both hands. Gently pull left leg toward chest. Stretches left hamstring and right hip flexor. Switch legs and repeat.

### Modified Hurdler's Stretch

Sit down, extend right leg and place left foot against inner right thigh. Gently bend forward from the hips, toward toes. Stretches the hamstring. Switch legs and repeat.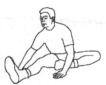

## Hip Stretch

Lie on back with knees bent, feet flat on the deck. Place right ankle on left knee. Grasp left thigh with both hands and gently pull it toward chest. Switch legs and repeat. Stretches hip extensors.

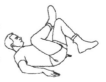

## Pretzel Stretch

Sit with both legs straight. Bend the left knee and cross left foot over the right shin. Turn torso left and place right elbow just below the left knee. Turn as far left as possible. Stretches hip abductors, lower back, and iliotibial band. Switch legs and repeat.

## Butterflies

Sit with legs bent and bottoms of feet together. Wrap hands around ankles and gently lean your torso forward, keeping your back flat. Do not pull on ankles or press knees down with elbows. Stretches hip adductors.

## Lunge

With feet side by side, take a large step forward with left foot. Bend your left knee until it is directly over left ankle. Gently press your hips forward and down, keeping your back straight. Stretches hip flexors. Switch legs and repeat.

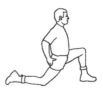

## Lizard

Lie face down, palms on the deck under your shoulders. Gently lift torso with arms and lower back muscles. Lift only until your pelvis is off the deck. Stretches the abdominals.

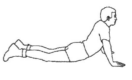

## Lower Back Stretch

Lie on back, bring knees to chest and grasp knees with hands (arms may either be below or above lower legs). Gently pull both knees toward chest. Lift chin toward chest. Stretches the lower back.

## Kneeling Back Stretch

Kneel down with knees shoulder width apart. Sit back on your heels. Lean forward so your chest rests on your thighs. Extend arms over head. Stretch arms and chest as far forward as possible. Stretches lower back.

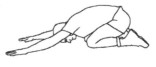

## Upper Back Stretch

Clasp hands together in front of chest, palms facing out, arms extended. Press through palms until back and shoulders are rounded. Stretches back and shoulders. Can do seated or standing.

## Posterior Shoulder Stretch

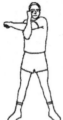

Bring left arm across chest. Use right hand to gently push upper left arm toward chest. Stretches shoulders. Switch arms and repeat.

## Triceps Stretch

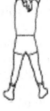

Bring left arm up and back until left palm is between shoulder blades and left elbow is above left ear. Gently grasp upper left arm with right hand and push left arm behind head. Stretches the triceps. Switch arms and repeat.

## Chest Stretch

Clasp hands behind lower back, thumbs pointed down. Gently pull arms up toward ceiling. Stretches chest and shoulders. Can do seated or standing.

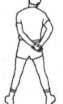

## Neck Stretch

Clasp hands behind back. Bend neck so right ear moves to right shoulder. Gently pull left arm. Stretches neck. Switch arms to stretch the right side of the neck.

## Table 9-2. Dynamic Stretches

### Neck Stretch

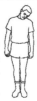

Begin from a standing position. Count 1: slowly roll the head to one side, Count 2: slowly roll the head to the front, Count 3: slowly roll the head to the other side, Count 4: slowly roll the head to the front again. Repeat. Do not roll the head back. Stretches the neck muscles. Variation: Turn your head to look over your right shoulder then slowly turn your head to look over your left shoulder. Repeat.

### Up Back and Over

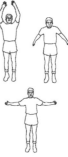

Begin from standing position with arms at sides. Count 1: slowly bring both arms forward and upward. Count 2: slowly bring both arms down and back. Count 3: slowly move both arms forward, up, back, and around to complete a full circle. Stretches the shoulders, chest, and back.

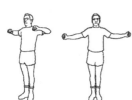

### Press-Press-Fling

Begin from a standing position with arms bent, fists at chest level, and elbows out to the side. Count 1: gently pull elbows back and release. Count 2: repeat count 1. Count 3: slowly extend arms and pull them back. Stretches the chest and shoulders.

### Trunk Twisters

Begin in a seated position with legs crossed and hands placed behind your head. Count 1: slowly turn your torso, at the waist, to the right and pause. Count 2: slowly turn your torso to the left and pause. Repeat. Stretches abdominals and obliques.

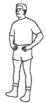

### Standing Toe Pointers

Start from a standing position with body weight over the heels. Flex and extend the feet and toes. Stretches both the calf muscles and the muscles in front of the shins. Variation: walk on the heels with toes pointed upward.

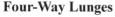

### Four-Way Lunges

Begin from a standing position. Count 1: lunge forward with right leg, distributing body weight across both legs. When lunging forward, the knee should not extend beyond the toe of that leg. Count 2: using the right leg, push off and return to start position. Repeat this movement using the same leg but lunge to the side. Perform exercise with the left leg. Stretches the leg muscles.

Table 9-1 and Table 9-2 were adapted from The Navy SEAL Physical Fitness Guide.

71

# 10 | Training in Confined Spaces

In this chapter you will learn about:

♦ Exercises to perform when space and equipment are limited.

♦ Designing a circuit training workout.

♦ Maintaining morale during deployment.

During deployment or extended training exercises you may encounter conditions that limit your physical training routines and options. Submarines and small assault craft probably create the greatest challenge, but a well balanced training program can be maintained even with limited space and equipment. So, take this opportunity to design new routines with alternative exercises and have fun. The concepts for designing training routines in confined spaces is the same as any gym-based routine, you just have to be more creative. Follow the FITT Principle guidelines outlined in Chapters 4, 5, and 7 and try some of the exercise in this chapter when designing your workouts.

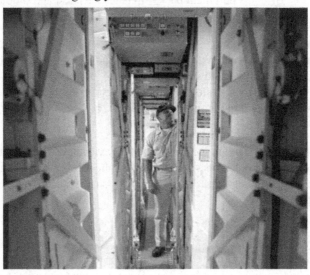

# Aerobic Conditioning

Some exercises for aerobic conditioning that you can perform in confined quarters with minimal equipment include:

♦ Jogging or marching in place.

♦ Jumping rope or jumping jacks

♦ Stair stepping, if you have access to stairs or if you have space for an aerobic step bench (plastic step with risers).

# Strength Training

Besides calisthenics, strength exercises with light-weight, portable equipment, such as elastic tubing, dumbbells or a ball, can be performed in small spaces. Examples of these exercises are shown in Table 10-1. Regardless of the equipment used, the general principles and techniques outlined in Chapter 7 for muscle strength and endurance training apply. Follow the set and rep recommendations outlined in Chapter 8 for calisthenic exercises, starting with one set of eight reps. Include exercises for each of the major muscle groups mentioned in Chapter 7, Figure 7-2.

## Elastic Tubing and Bands

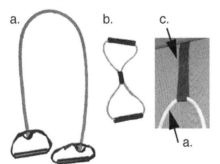

a. 4 ft. elastic band.

b. 1 ft. elastic loop with foam handles.

c. Nylon anchor piece to place in door jams.

These come in different widths and resistances, each designated by a different color. (As a rule, the smaller the tube's width, the less resistance it provides.) The basis of elastic tubing exercises is that as you stretch the tubing during your exercise, it provides a continuously increasing resistance. Resistance can be adjusted by: 1) altering the placement of the tubing (addressed in Table 10-1), 2) using two tubes, 3) using a thicker tube, or a combination of all these. Note that using two thin tubes may provide less resistance than using one thick tube. Typically, tubes and bands are sold in 4 ft. lengths and cost $5 to $10. When purchasing tubing, buy one with handles large enough to slip over your forearms. Buy several tubes of varying widths since you will need different resistances for different exercises. Also, check the tubes periodically for wear and tear.

73

## Inflatable Resistance Balls

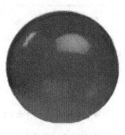

These light-weight balls are becoming very popular in fitness centers and are excellent for abdominal, lower back, stability, and stretching exercises. The goal in resistance ball training is to keep your balance and stability while performing exercises on the ball, which acts as an unstable base. Resistance balls are typically 18 to 30 inches in diameter and cost about $30. Purchase a resistance ball that when you sit on it after it is fully inflated, your thighs are parallel to the deck. In addition, when you purchase these balls, you get a video of various exercises and routines. One drawback is that you need access to an air pump because, if the ball is kept inflated, it can take up a lot of storage space.

## Strength Exercises

Table 10-1 shows exercises that can be performed using resistance tubing (bands) and balls. When performing elastic tubing exercises, you can use a partner, instead of an anchor, to secure the tubing during your exercise. Just be sure your partner holds the tubing at the appropriate height and distance from you (and doesn't let go!). When using the resistance bands, it is important to anchor them properly. Some examples are shown in Figure 10-1.

## Figure 10-1. Anchoring Elastic Tubing

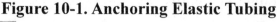

1. 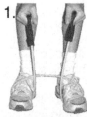 1. Wrap the band around the top and sides of both feet, then pull the handles up through the middle of your feet.This type of wrap is useful for anchoring the band during rowing exercises.

2. 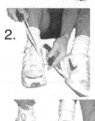 2. a.  Using the 1 ft. elastic loop, sit down and place your right foot on the middle of the loop.
b.    Wrap the right end of the tubing over your foot.
c.    Pull the left end of the tubing up through the right end of the tubing loop.
d.    Take the left end of the tubing loop and wrap it around your left foot. This type of anchor is useful for leg lifts and leg curls.

Table 10-1. Exercises to Perform in Confined Spaces

# Back

### Bent-Over Row with Band

Grab one end of the band in each hand. Step on the middle of the band with your left foot, step back 2 ft. with your right foot. Bend forward slightly at the waist, keep your shoulders and hips facing forward. Count 1: Lift both hands from your thighs to your waist. This should take 2 seconds. Pause for 1 second. Count 2: Return hands to thigh level in 4 seconds. Keep your elbows close to your body throughout the exercise. Works the back and biceps muscles.

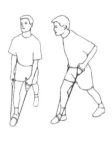

### Lat Pull down with Band

Secure the middle of the band to a fixed object above your head. Grasp one handle in each hand. Facing the anchor, step back 1 foot and kneel. Arms should be extended above head. Count 1: Pull hands down to shoulder height in front of your head, keeping chest and head up. Back should remain straight. Press your shoulder blades together in the middle of your back as you pull your arms down. This should take 2 seconds. Pause 1 second. Count 2: Return to start position in 4 seconds. Variation: may need to use the tubing loop instead of a band for adequate resistance.

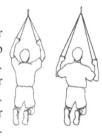

### Seated Row with Band

Sit on deck with legs extended, knees slightly bent. Place the center of the band under your feet. Count 1: With arms extended at chest level and hands over knees, bend your elbows and pull your hands back to each side of your chest. This should take 2 seconds. Pause 1 second. Count 2; Return to start position in 4 seconds. Works back and biceps.

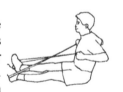

# Lower Back

### Lower Back on Ball

Kneel beside resistance ball, lay your chest on top of the ball, place your hands in front of the ball. Extend your legs so only your feet are on the deck and walk forward, rolling the ball back closer to your hips. Place your hands behind your back. Count 1: Keep your back straight and raise your torso up off the ball until your back is extended. Count 2: Return to the start position. Try to keep ball steady during exercise. Works the lower back. Similar to prone back extension performed on the deck. Variations: Can do all the same extension exercises as on the deck.

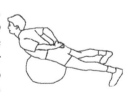

## Abdominals

### Abdominal Crunch with Band

Anchor the middle of the band above your head. Kneel 1 ft. in front of the anchor, and grasp both ends of the band in your hands. Place your hands palms down on your shoulders. Count 1: Pull your rib cage down closer to your hips. This should take 2 seconds. Pause 1 second. Keep your hips and legs still. Count 2: Return to the start position in 4 seconds.

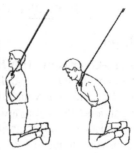

### Abdominal Crunch on Ball

Sit on ball, slowly walk feet away from ball as you lie back on to the ball. Ball should be underneath your midback. Place your hands behind your head. Count 1: Pull your rib cage closer to your hips. Count 2: Return to the start position. Try to keep ball steady during exercise. Works the abdominals. Variations: Use a towel under your lower back instead of the ball; perform side crunches on the ball to target the obliques.

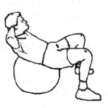

### Table 10-1. Exercises to Perform in Confined Spaces

## Chest

### Chest Fly with Band

Sit on the deck with your left leg straight and your right leg bent, with your right foot touching your left thigh. Hold one handle of the band in each hand. Wrap the band under your left heel, about 1/3 the length of the band down from your left hand. Keep your back straight, head up, and shoulders back. Place your right hand on the deck by your right knee. Straighten your left arm so that your elbow is only slightly bent and raise your arm in front of you to chest level. Count 1: Slowly pull your upper left arm across your chest without bending your elbow; this should take 2 seconds. Pause for 1 second. Count 2: Return to the start position in 4 seconds. Your torso and hips

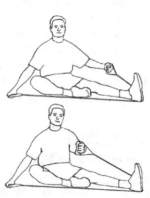

should not move during this exercise. Works your chest muscles. Variations: a) perform this standing or kneeling by anchoring the band to a stationary object at chest height; b) lie on your back on a bench and use dumbbells; c) have a partner push (manual resistance) against your upper arms as you do the exercise.

# Chest Press with Band

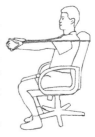

Wrap the band at shoulder height around a bench that is wider than shoulder-width (or secure with two anchors). Keep your back straight, shoulders down and head up. Grip one end of the band in each hand, and place your hands on each side of your chest. Count 1: Extend arms straight in frontof you at chest height, do not lock your elbows; this should take 2 seconds. Pause for 1 second. Count 2: Return to the start position in 4 seconds. Works your chest, shoulders, and triceps.Variations: a) have a partner hold the band in both hands, keeping his hands at your shoulder height and wider than your shoulder-width; b) lie on back on a bench and use dumbbells; c) have a partner provide manual resistance against your hands as you perform a press.

### Incline Press with Band

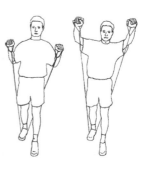

Grab one end of the band in each hand. Step on the band with your right foot, step your left foot through the band and forward 2 ft. Bring your hands to your shoulders with your palms facing forward. Count 1: Extend your arms up and forward in front; your hands should be in front of and a little higher than your forehead. This should take 2 seconds. Pause for 1 second. Count 2: Return to start position. Works the chest and shoulders. Variations: a) for more resistance, use a second tube and place it under your front foot; b) for less resistance, anchor the tube to a stationary object at waist height, step forward 2 ft. and perform the exercise.

## Biceps

### Biceps Curl with Band

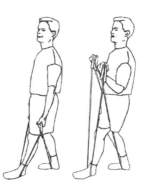

Grab one end of the band in each your chest. Count 1: Extend arms straight in front of you at chest height, do not lock your elbows; this should take 2 seconds. Pause for 1 second. second. Count 2: Return to start Count 2: Return to the start position in 4 seconds. position. Works the biceps. Works your chest, shoulders, and triceps. Variations: a) have a partner hold the band in both hands, keeping his hands at your shoulder height and wider than your shoulder-width; b) lie on back on a bench and use dumbbells; c) have a partner provide manual resistance against your hands as you perform a press. Variations: a) for more resistance, use a second tube (as shown) and place it under your front foot); b) use dumbbells; c) have a partner pull against your lower arm during the curl.

**Table 10-1. Exercises to Perform in Confined Spaces**

## Triceps

### Triceps Extension with Band

Stand with feet hip distance apart, knees slightly bent. Grab one end of the band in your right hand and place it over your right shoulder. Your right elbow should be beside your head and the band should be dangling down your back. Reach around your back with your left hand and grab the other end of the band with your left hand. Place your left hand on your low back. Count 1: Extend your right arm straight above your head, keeping your left hand still and your right elbow close to your head. Do not lock your right elbow. This should take 2 seconds. Pause 1 second. Count 2: Return to the start

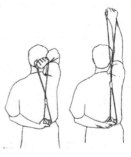

position in 4 seconds. Works the right triceps. Switch arms to work the left triceps. Variations: a) if you have a long piece of tubing, grab the middle of the tubing (instead of the end) with your left hand; b) use dumbbells

### Triceps Kickback with Band

Grab one end of the band in each hand. Step on the middle of the band with your left foot, step back 2 ft. with your right foot. Bend forward slightly at the waist, keep your shoulders and hips facing forward. Place your left hand on your left thigh for support. Pull your right hand up to your right hip, keeping your right elbow close to your body. Count 1: Straighten your lower right arm behind your back without lifting your elbow. This should take 2 seconds. Pause 1

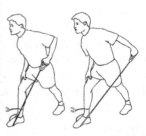

second. Count 2: Return to the start position in 4 seconds. Works the right triceps. Switch to work the left triceps. Variations: a) use dumbbells; b) have a partner push against your lower arm during the lift.

## Shoulders

### Lateral Raise with Band

Grab one end of the band in each hand. Stand on middle of the band, feet shoulder-width apart, knees slightly bent. With arms at sides, bend elbows 90o. Count 1: raise your upper arms to each side until your elbow (still bent 90o) is level with your shoulder. This should take 2 seconds. Pause 1 second. Count 2: Return to start position in 4 seconds. Keep your elbow bent during the lift. Works the shoulders. Variations: a) for more resistance, use 2 bands, stand on only one band with

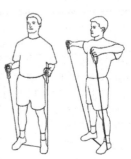

each foot, hold one end of each band in each hand; b) use dumbbells; c) have a partner push down against your upper arms as you lift; d) increase the difficulty of the exercise by straightening your elbow.

### Upright Rows with Band

Stand on the middle of the band, feet shoulder-width apart, knees slightly bent. Cross ends of band in front of you and grasp one end of the band in each hand, palms facing back. Count 1: With arms extended and hands together at the center of your body, pull elbows up and back to the level of your shoulders. Your arms should form a "V". This should take 2 seconds. Pause 1 second. Count 2: Return to start position in 4 seconds. Do not arch your back during the lift. Works the front of the shoulders. Variations: a) for more resistance, use 2 bands, stand on only one band with each foot, hold one end of each band in each hand; b) use dumbbells.

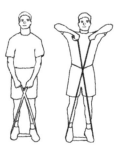

### Reverse Fly with Band

Anchor the middle of the band at chest height. Facing the anchor, step back 4-5 ft. Grab one end of the band in each hand. Extend your arms straight in front of you at chest level, elbows slightly bent. Count 1: Pull your upper arms out to each side without bending your elbows any more. This should take 2 seconds. Pause 1 second. Count 2: Return to the start position in 4 seconds. Works the back of the shoulders. Variations: a) kneel on one knee, bend at the waist, rest chest on opposite thigh, and use dumbbells or have a partner push against your upper arms.

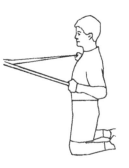

## Legs

### Lunge with Band

Grab one end of the band in each hand. Step on the middle of the band with your left foot, step your right foot through the band and beside your left foot. Bring hands up to shoulders, palms facing forward. Band should be behind your arms. Count 1: Take a large step forward with your right foot, keep your back straight and head up. Count 2: Squat straight down, dropping your left knee, until your right knee is over your right ankle. Count 3: Lift up. Count 4: Push off your right foot to return to the start position. Works the leg muscles.

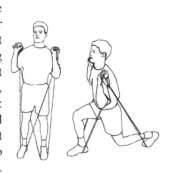

Switch sides. Variation: a) for more resistance, use a second tube and place it under your front foot; b) on Count 1, step to the left or right instead of straight ahead; c) use dumbbells.

### Leg Curl with Band

Wrap one end of the tubing loop around your right foot. Hook the other end on your left foot. Lie on your stomach with both legs extended. Count 1: Lift your left heel up toward your buttocks, keeping your right knee and hips flat on the deck. This should take 2 seconds. Pause 1 second. Count 2: Lower your leg to the start position in 4 seconds. Works the hamstrings.

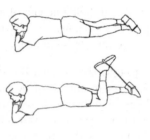

### Leg Lifts with Band

Anchor the band at shin height. Wrap the band around your left ankle and, facing the anchor, step back 3 ft. Place feet side by side and point your left foot up. Place your hand on the wall for support and slightly bend your right knee. Count 1: Keeping your left leg extended, pull your left ankle back 1-2 ft. This should take 2 seconds. Pause for 1 second. Count 2: Return to start position in 4 seconds. Switch legs. Works hamstring and gluteal muscles. Variations: a) to work inner and outer thighs and hip flexors, change the position of your body so you pull against the band in all four directions (front, back, and two sides); b) lie down and use ankle weights.

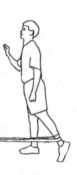

### Squat with Band

Grasp one handle in each hand, step on the band with feet hip-width apart, knees slightly bent. Bring hands up to shoulders, palms facing forward. Band should be behind your arms. Count 1: Slowly squat down; look forward, keeping your shoulders back, chest and head up. Squat until your knees are above your toes. This should take 2 seconds. Pause 1 second. Count 2: Return to the start position in 4 seconds. Works the quadriceps and gluteals.

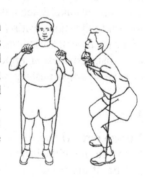

### Wall Squat with Ball

Stand against a flat wall, place both feet 2 ft. from the wall hip distance apart. Place a small ball between your knees. Count 1: Slide down the wall until your knees are over your feet and squeeze the ball between your knees. Hold this position for 10 seconds. Count 2: Return to the start position. Works the thigh muscles. Variations: a) hold dumbbells in your hands.

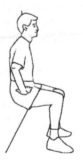

# Workout Design

Since space, equipment, and time are limiting factors during deployment, one of the most effective workouts for you to perform is circuit training (described in Chapter 7). The basics of this type of workout are:

♦ Total session is 30-60 minutes, divided into 30-60 second stations.

♦ Each station is a new exercise; alternate aerobic and strength stations, and upper and lower body exercises.

♦ Perform aerobic exercises in your target heart rate zone.

♦ Perform strength exercises with proper form and use a resistance that you can lift 10-12 times.

♦ Stretch after your workout. (See Chapter 9.)

When designing a circuit training routine, follow the FITT principle guidelines outlined in Chapters 4, 5, and 7.

## Table 10-2. Circuit Training Workout

| Station | Exercise | Time |
|---------|----------|------|
| | Warm-up | 5 minutes |
| 1 | Wall Squat with Ball | 60 sec |
| 2 | Push ups | 60 sec |
| 3 | Jog in place | 60 sec |
| 4 | Stair step/Jog | 60 sec |
| 5 | Jumping Jacks | 60 sec |
| | Check heart rate | 10 sec |
| 6 | Lat Pulldown with Band | 60 sec |
| 7 | Abdominal Crunches and Lower Back Extensions | 60 sec (30 sec each) |
| 8 | Biceps curl and Triceps Extension with band | 60 sec (30 sec each) |
| 9 | Jumping Jacks | 60 sec |
| 10 | Stair Step/Jog | 60 sec |
| 11 | Jog in place | 60 sec |
| 12 | Jumping Jacks | 60 sec |
| | Check heart rate | 10 sec |
| | Repeat Stations 1-12, 2-4 times | |
| | Cool Down | 5 minutes |
| | Stretch | 5-10 minutes |

Note: One cycle of this circuit training workout has 7 minutes of aerobic exercises and one set of strength exercises for each of the major muscle groups.

# Morale During Deployment

Although confined spaces can limit your training options and make you feel less than enthusiastic to train, you need to remain physically active. Stopping all physical training results in a rapid decline in muscle strength and endurance, flexibility, and aerobic conditioning (see Chapter 4). One option to boost morale and increase participation in physical 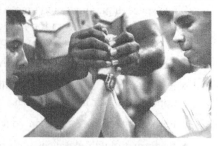 training during deployment is to help organize and participate in team competitions such as mini-triathlons (perform any three aerobic exercises back-to-back for the best time) and sports days.

Finally, you may feel that the biggest barrier to working out when deployed is time limitations. In actuality, it requires less time to maintain fitness levels than to increase fitness levels. Though not ideal, you can maintain your fitness level by working at your usual intensity fewer times per week and for shorter durations than what is required to improve your fitness level. A minimum of one strength session, which includes exercises for all the major muscle groups (1 set of 8-12 repetitions), and two 20-minute aerobic sessions, within your target heart rate zone, per week will allow you to maintain your current fitness level. Though this limited amount of training is not ideal for your overall fitness, it is much better than not performing any exercise at all. Remember, detraining occurs rapidly when all training is stopped (see Chapter 4).

# 11 |  Nutrition for Exercise

In this chapter you will learn about:

♦ Dietary practices for enhancing endurance and strength performance.

♦ Dietary measures for exercise recovery.

Your physical performance is greatly influenced by regular conditioning and by following sound dietary practices. Both prolonged aerobic exercise and multiple bouts of high intensity exercise impose significant demands on energy and fluid balance. Failure to replace energy and fluids used during exercise can significantly impair performance in later activities.

The following recommendations are for an individual who regularly participates in at least 90 minutes of aerobic exercise each day or in multiple, strenuous bouts of exercise several times a week. This information does not apply if you exercise less than one hour per day.

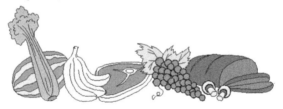

## Carbohydrate Needs

During heavy training you must increase your kcal intake, especially from carbohydrates (CHO), to meet your energy demands. Failure to do so may result in:

♦ Chronic muscular fatigue.

♦ A feeling of staleness.

♦ Weight and muscle mass loss.

### CHO for Endurance Training

The endurance capacity of an individual on a high-CHO diet is approximately **3 times greater** than on a high-fat diet. When CHO intake is low, several days of rigorous training will deplete muscle CHO (glycogen) stores and eventually impair performance. **CHO should supply 60 -65% of your total daily kcal intake**. Keep a dietary log for a few days to see if your CHO intake is adequate.

## Worksheet 11-1. Calculate Your Daily CHO Needs

_____ x 0.60 = _____ kcal from CHO per day.
Your EER*

_____ x 0.65 = _____ kcal from CHO per day.
Your EER*

You should eat _____ to _____ kcals from CHO daily.

\* Your estimated energy requirement (EER) was calculated in Chapter 1, Worksheet 1-2. To calculate grams of CHO see Worksheet 2-1.

## CHO Loading

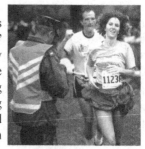

CHO Loading, or glycogen supercompensation, is a regimen that combines diet and exercise to "pack" more CHO (glycogen) into muscle. It is used by endurance athletes to optimize physical performance during prolonged endurance events. CHO loading is unnecessary for individuals who eat according to the dietary guidelines outlined in Chapter 3 and whose CHO intakes are within the range calculated in Worksheet 11-1.

## CHO for Strength Training

CHO are required for strength training because the exercises rely on muscle glycogen stores for energy. **CHO should supply 55-60% of your total daily caloric intake**. This is slightly lower than the requirements for endurance activities (see Worksheet 11-1) because the total amount of energy endurance activities (see Worksheet 11-1) because the total amount of energy expended is less.

# Protein Needs

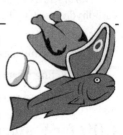

Protein needs of strength athletes and endurance athletes are quite similar at **0.6 - 0.8 grams of proteins per pound of body weight**.

This corresponds roughly to 10-15% of your total daily kcals. It is highly likely that your diet provides adequate proteins since most Americans consume proteins in excess of their needs. Use Worksheet 11-2 or Worksheet 2-2 (Chapter 2) to determine your protein needs.

## Worksheet 11-2. Calculate Your Protein Needs

Body Weight = _____ lbs.

0.6 grams/lb x _____ lbs. = _____ grams proteins.
             (Body weight)

0.8 grams/lb x _____ lbs. = _____ grams proteins.
             (Body weight)

Your daily protein grams = _____ to _____.

## The High-Protein Myth

One of the most common myths is that eating high-protein diets and protein supplements leads to bigger muscles. Clearly, this is not the case! Muscle is only 20%

Muscle is:
  20% proteins,
  75% water, and
  5% inorganic salts, urea,
    and lactate.

proteins; the rest is water, minerals, lactic acid, and urea. Moreover, excessive protein intakes, mostly from protein supplements, can cause:

♦ Increased water needs.

♦ Greater demands on the liver and the kidneys.

♦ Imbalances in the essential amino acids.

♦ Diarrhea or abdominal cramps.

For these reasons, avoid protein powder drinks that provide excessive amounts of proteins or selected amino acids. Supplements can be very expensive, dangerous to your health, and they are quite unnecessary. Spend your money on a variety of foods for a balanced diet that will sufficiently meet your protein needs. Exercise to gain muscle!

# Vitamin and Mineral Needs

Any increased vitamin and mineral needs can be met by eating according to the Food Guide Pyramid (Chapter 3, Figure 3-1). Particularly, increase the number of fruits and vegetables you eat as these foods are good sources of many vitamins and minerals, as well as antioxidants (see Chapter 3, Table 2-2, Table 2-3, and Appendix A). Antioxidant (see Glossary) nutrients may protect you from environmental stressors and may accelerate your recovery from exhaustive exercise. Fresh fruits and vegetables also provide potassium, which is lost during prolonged strenuous exercise (see Table 2-3).

# Fluid Needs

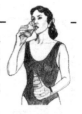

Drinking fluids at regular intervals and eating foods with a high water content (i.e., fresh fruits) are important for maintaining hydration and fluid status during training. See Chapter 2 for more information on fluid balance. Guidelines for drinking fluids during exercise are:

♦ Drink 16 oz. (2 cups) of fluid two hours before starting exercise.

♦ Drink 3 to 4 oz. (1/2 cup) of fluid every 15-20 minutes during exercise.

♦ Weigh yourself before and after exercise. Drink 16 oz. of fluid for every pound of weight lost.

♦ Do not rely on thirst as an indicator of fluid needs. Once you feel thirsty you are already dehydrated.

♦ Drink water when exercising less than 60 minutes. Drink a sports drink (5% to 8% CHO with electrolytes) when exercising longer than 60 minutes.

♦ Monitor your urine: urine should be a pale yellow and you should be urinating frequently.

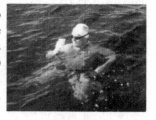

Many beverages can replenish lost fluids, so select a beverage that tastes good, does not cause stomach discomfort, is rapidly absorbed, and contains electrolytes (see Glossary) and CHO (5% to 8%) when performing prolonged or strenuous exercise. Rehydrate with a non-caffeinated, non-carbonated, non-alcoholic beverage.

## Overhydration

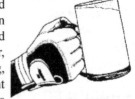

Although less common than dehydration, untreated overhydration can be life threatening. It is seen when plain water is used to replace fluid losses during prolonged (greater than 3 hours) strenuous exercise. Remember, both water and electrolytes are lost during sweating, so both need to be replaced in this situation. Prevent overhydration by drinking a beverage that contains electrolytes (such as a sport drink) or by eating a light snack (e.g., oranges) with your water. Between exercise sessions, electrolytes lost through sweating can be easily replaced by eating well-balanced meals and snacks (Chapter 3).

# Nutrition for Exercise Recovery

Within 30 minutes of completing an extended or intense exercise session, consume at least **50 grams of CHO** (roughly 200 kcals). Also, continue to snack on high-CHO foods for up to six hours. This will help restore your muscle glycogen (CHO stores) for the next exercise session. Some foods and servings sizes that contain roughly 50 grams of CHO are:

♦ Bagel with jam

♦ Baked potato with skin

♦ Cooked sweet corn, 1.5 cups

♦ Cornflakes, 2.5 cups

♦ Watermelon, 4.5 cups

♦ Raisins, 0.4 cup

♦ Shredded wheat cereal, 1.4 cups

♦ Baked Beans, 1 cup

♦ Bananas (2)

♦ Cooked oatmeal, 2 cups

♦ Cooked Rice, 1 cup

♦ Orange juice, 2 cups

For more information on the CHO content of foods, check food labels (Figure 3-2), check the USDA website at http://www.usda.gov, or ask a dietitian.

# 12 | Deployment and Altered Climates

In this chapter you will learn about:

♦ Acclimation.

♦ General guidelines for altered environments.

♦ Maintaining performance in the heat, cold, and at altitude.

Adapting, or acclimating, to a new environment, such as extreme changes in climate or altitude, imposes considerable demands on the body. Proper acclimation is necessary in order for the body to function more efficiently in a new environment.

## Acclimating to Altered Environments

Adapting to a new environment (e.g., heat, cold, altitude) can take one to three weeks. Having a good aerobic fitness base will accelerate your acclimation to new environments. However, factors that can negatively affect acclimation include:

♦ Dehydration.

♦ Drinking alcohol.

♦ Cessation of physical activity

♦ Electrolyte depletion.

♦ Inadequate energy intake.

♦ Illness.

♦ Infection.

♦ Injury.

♦ Loss of sleep.

General guidelines for nutrition and physical activity in altered climates are outlined and followed by brief descriptions of the effects that heat, cold, and altitude have on metabolism.

## General Nutrition Issues

Adapting to adverse environments increases energy expenditure and water losses. If energy and fluid needs are not met then performance will decline. Consult a registered dietitian if you have questions about your nutrient requirements. Strategies to maintain energy and fluid balance are:

## Meeting Energy Needs

- ♦ Eat a high-CHO diet (roughly 60% of your total daily kcals) to meet increased kcal needs.

- ♦ Keep fat intakes to less than 30% of your total daily kcals.

- ♦ Keep protein intakes to about 10% of your total daily kcals. Also, avoid amino acid and protein supplements (see Chapter 2).

- ♦ Eat small frequent meals.

- ♦ Eat all components of your field rations.

## Meeting Fluid Needs

Maintaining fluid balance is crucial to avoid dehydration (Chapter 2). Dehydration can limit performance and severe dehydration can be life-threatening. Tips for maintaining fluid balance include:

- ♦ Monitor hydration status (Chapter 11).

- ♦ Monitor fluid status by weighing yourself prior to and after prolonged physical activities. Drink 2 cups (0.45 L or 16 oz.) of water for every pound of body weight lost.

- ♦ Thirst is not a good indicator of fluid status. Drink fluids regularly throughout the day. When working in the heat, do not drink more than 6 cups of fluid an hour.

- ♦ When exercising or working for prolonged periods (>60 minutes), drink a fluid replacement beverage such as a sports drink instead of water (see Chapter 11).

- ♦ Avoid alcoholic beverages; alcohol increases fluid losses.

- ♦ Reduce caffeine consumption; caffeine increases fluid losses.

- ♦ Avoid salty foods; salt increases fluid needs.

# Physical Activity Concerns

General considerations for physical work and exercising in environmental extremes include:

- ♦ Plan for decreased physical performance the first two weeks.

- ♦ Plan your workouts to avoid the hottest or coldest times of the day and allow adequate time for warm-ups.

- ♦ Drink plenty of fluids and eat enough kcals to replace lost fluids, CHO, and electrolytes.

- ♦ Be aware of conditions that may predispose you to dehydration (diarrhea, vomiting, fever). Also, avoid substances that can lead to dehydration such as caffeine and alcohol.

# Hot Environments

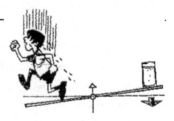

When the temperature and humidity are over 85° F and 60%, respectively exercise should be performed indoors or undertaken with caution. Any time you perform physical activities in the heat, you will lose a lot of water and minerals through sweat. Although appetites may be suppressed in the hot weather, adequate caloric intake is important. Energy requirements can increase by 10% in order to maintain a normal body temperature

**If your activity level decreases, you don't need extra kcals!**

# Cold Environments

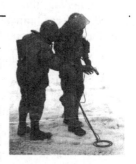

It is considered cold if the air temperature is below 15° F and the wind speed is greater than 25 m.p.h, or the water temperature is below 64°F. Cold environments increase energy metabolism and urination.

Soldiers can progressively lose weight when conducting field exercises in the cold for two to three weeks. Because this weight loss can cause fatigue and performance decrements, energy intake must increase to meet the increased energy demands. Energy requirements can increase 25 to 50% in the cold. To meet the increased energy and fluid needs, follow the guidelines. Also, vitamin and mineral needs may increase, so eat all ration components to meet these needs.

# Altitude

Ascent to altitude can cause a variety of physiologic disturbances due to the drops in temperature and humidity, and the lack of oxygen. Some major concerns are weight loss, disturbances in digestion, nutrient and fluid needs, and Acute Mountain Sickness (AMS). Adequate nutrition can play a crucial role in maintaining health and performance at altitude.

Energy requirements are 15-50% greater at altitude than at sea level. Virtually everyone who goes to higher altitudes experiences weight loss and loss of muscle mass. At altitudes below 5,000 m weight loss can be prevented by increasing your kcal intakes. Weight loss is inevitable above 5,000 m. To meet the increased energy and fluid needs at altitude follow the guidelines.

Vitamin and mineral needs are likely to increase at altitude. In particular, the increased metabolic rate and the lack of oxygen can increase the production of harmful free radicals. Preliminary research indicates that taking 400 IU per day of vitamin E, an antioxidant, at high altitude reduces free radical production.

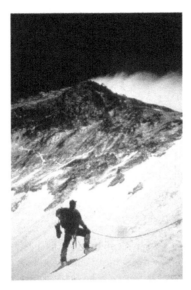

As noted throughout this chapter, meeting energy and fluid requirements are vital to maintain physical performance in adverse environmental conditions. Being physically fit and eating a healthy diet prior to deployment will greatly improve your adaptation to the new environment.

# 13 | Training and Overuse Injuries

In this chapter you will learn about:

♦ Treatment and prevention of injuries.

♦ When to seek medical care.

♦ Returning to duty.

♦ Overtraining syndrome.

One of the hazards of physical training is becoming injured. Sustaining either a sudden injury or an overuse injury can mean loss of work days, forced rest, and pain for a period of days to weeks. The goal of this chapter is not to have you treat your own injuries, but rather to be informed so that you will seek appropriate help when needed.

## Injuries: Treatment and Prevention

A variety of injuries can occur during physical training. Table 13-1 has a brief description of acute and overuse injuries, as well as their treatment and prevention.

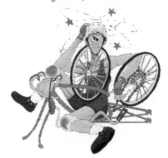

The treatment of any injury should focus on controlling inflammation and allowing full joint range of motion for a rapid return to daily activities.

## Table 13-1. Injuries, Treatments, and Prevention

| Injury | Treatment | Prevention |
|---|---|---|
| **Delayed-Onset Muscle Soreness** - Muscle pain occurring in deconditioned muscle 12 to 72+ hours after training. | Ice, stretch, warm-up. Do not use NSAIDs. | Resolves as muscle adapts to training. Slowly increase training intensity. |
| **Contusions** - Swelling and bleeding (bruising) in the muscle, tendon, or bone due to a direct blow. | Ice | Wear protective gear. |
| **Muscle Cramp** - Muscle pain caused by prolonged activity, high heat or humidity, dehydration, and poor conditioning. | Rehydrate (Chapter 2), stretch, massage with ice. | Allow time to adjust to training and climate; drink frequently. |
| **True Fractures** - Break or chip in the bone. | Seek medical help. | Use protective gear; recondition. |
| **Stress Fractures** - Pain and weakening of the bone caused by excessive stress and use. | Seek medical help. | Reduce high-impact activities, cross-train, use proper gear, slowly increase training. |
| **Sprains** - Acute or overuse injury to ligaments (connective tissue that joins bone to bone). | RICE.* Seek medical help. | Follow medical advise; slowly increase training intensity, use proper gear. |
| **Strains, Tendonitis** - Acute or overuse injury to muscle or tendons (connective tissue that joins muscle to bone). | RICE. Seek medical help. | See "Sprains." |
| **Heat Injuries (cramp, exhaustion, heat stroke)** - Painful muscle contractions, nausea, fatigue, fever, or dizziness from dehydration and electrolyte depletion; fevers >104°F can damage vital organs and result in death. | Place person in a cool location and rehydrate. Seek medical help. | Acclimate to climate, avoid exercise in extreme heat, avoid substances that cause dehydration (Chapter 12), stay well hydrated (Chapter 2). |
| **Cold Injuries (hypothermia, frost bite, trench foot)** - Body temperature <95°F causing shivers, slurred speech, clumsiness, and freezing of exposed body parts. | Gently place the person in dry blankets with another warm person. | Wear proper gear, stay dry, avoid exercise in extreme cold, stay well hydrated (Chapter 2). |

RICE = rest, ice, compression, and elevation; See page 78.

To accelerate healing, you must first decrease the inflammatory process. Treatment steps to achieve this include:

### RICE = Rest + Ice + Compression + Elevation

♦ **Rest** - no weight-bearing of the injured limb, using crutches for locomotion.

♦ **Ice** - as soon as possible apply ice, wrapped in a bag or towel, to the injured area. Ice for 20 minutes every two hours on the first day, then 3 times a day until the swelling has decreased. Do not ice for longer than 20 minutes at a time. Never apply ice directly to the skin or to an open wound!

♦ **Compression** - wrap the injury for periods of 2 to 4 hours. Never sleep with a compression wrap unless medically advised.

♦ **Elevation** - place the injury above the level of the heart, allowing gravity to reduce the swelling.

## Non-Steroidal Anti-Inflammatory Drugs (NSAIDs)

In addition to RICE, non-steroidal anti-inflammatory drugs (NSAIDs) are often used. In the case of an acute injury which involves bleeding, bruising, or swelling, NSAIDs should not be started until after the bleeding has stopped (may take days) and the swelling has stabilized. Some side-effects of NSAIDs include:

♦ Nausea, heartburn, vomiting, ulcers, and bleeding.

♦ Increased blood pressure.

♦ Decreased ability of blood to clot.

♦ Worsening of asthma.

♦ Potential kidney damage with long-term use.

Some of the most common NSAIDs are aspirin (Bayer, Aspirin, Ecotrin), ibuprofen (Advil, Motrin), and ketoprofen (Orudis). NSAIDs should not be used with alcohol. If you have stomach or gastrointestinal problems, check with your doctor for the appropriate pain reliever.

### When to Seek Medical Care

Conditions that demand immediate medical attention include numbness, suspected fracture, joint dislocation, hip pain that causes a limp, pain that limits activity for more than 3 days, back pain that radiates into the leg and foot, and any lower extremity injury on which you cannot bear weight.

## Return to Duty

After the pain and swelling are reduced and full range of motion is possible, ask your physician or physical therapist to design a reconditioning exercise program with the overall goal of **returning to full activity**. The exercises prescribed will be specific to the site and type of injury.

## Overtraining Syndrome

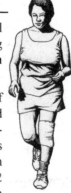

Overtraining can negatively affect physical and mental performance. Moreover, it can increase the likelihood of sustaining an injury. Overtraining is exactly what the word implies: **too much physical activity**.

The **overtraining syndrome** can present with a wide range of symptoms (See Table 13-2). Overtraining is generally associated with endurance sports, such as swimming or running. Cross-training, rest, and taking time off from certain physical activities will all reduce or prevent overtraining symptoms. The person who continues training despite the symptoms listed in Table 13-2 will only become more overtrained, continue to have decreases in performance, and will be at an increased risk for injury.

## Table 13-2. Symptoms of Overtraining Syndrome

♦ Decreased performance.

♦ Difficulty making decisions.

♦ Chronically fatigued.

♦ Lacking motivation.

♦ Disturbances in mood.

♦ Feeling depressed.

♦ Increased morning heart rate.

♦ Feeling "burned-out" or stale.

♦ Difficulty concentrating.

♦ Angry and irritable.

♦ Muscle soreness.

♦ Increased distractibility.

♦ Difficulty sleeping.

# 14 | Supplements and Performance

In this chapter you will learn about:

- ♦ Vitamin and mineral supplements.
- ♦ Nutritional ergogenic agents; hype versus reality.
- ♦ Risks associated with using performance enhancers.
- ♦ Ergolytic agents.

Gaining and maintaining physical fitness takes time and dedication. Often, to achieve these goals, people turn to various supplements based on their claims as performance enhancers. However, no supplement can replace the benefits of a well-planned exercise routine and a nutritionally-sound diet!

## Vitamin and Mineral Supplements

Taking a vitamin or mineral supplement may be something you are considering, especially if you find it difficult to eat a variety of foods. Due to the various functions of vitamins and minerals, the supplement industry has tried to encourage supplement use by physically active people. However, multivitamin and mineral supplements do not appear to enhance performance in healthy, well-nourished individuals. A multivitamin and mineral supplement is useful if:

- ♦ You have an existing vitamin or mineral deficiency.
- ♦ You have poor dietary habits. In this case, increase the amount of nutrient dense foods and food variety in your diet!
- ♦ You are exposed to extreme environmental conditions, such as cold climates or high altitudes (Chapter 12).

### Buying Vitamin and Mineral Supplements

- ♦ Some facts to know before buying a supplement are:
- ♦ Amount of Nutrients - Take a multi-vitamin and mineral supplement that supplies nutrients in amounts close to the RDA/DRIs (Chapter 2). Excessive amounts of a single nutrient can cause a deficiency of other nutrients. Avoid "high potency" supplements.
- ♦ Natural Versus Synthetic Vitamins - Both forms can be used by your body, but if a supplement is labelled

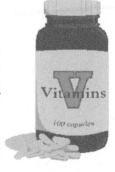

96

"natural" it costs more.

♦ Expiration Date - Avoid supplements that expire in 6 months.

♦ Stress tablets are a marketing ploy.

♦ Men should not take iron supplements, unless directed by their doctor.

# Nutritional Ergogenic Agents

Taking performance-enhancing supplements is a personal choice. Table 14-1 lists some popular ergogenic agents grouped by type (identified in bold), the research findings, and the potential side effects. However, this list is not complete as new supplements enter the market regularly. This table is designed to educate you as a consumer. Many of the ergogenic agents listed are classified as nutritional supplements. When marketed as a nutritional supplement, these substances are **not regulated by the Federal Drug Administration (FDA)**. Often this means that the performance claims and the risks associated with using these substances have not been thoroughly tested.

Other sources of information include the **Ergogenics Pamphlet** (http:// www. usuhs.mil/mim/ergopam.pdf); the Alcohol Tobacco and Firearms web site at http:// www.ATF.treas.gov; the Federal Drug Agency at http:// www.fda.gov (select the "Food" icon); and the Federal Trade Commission at http://www.ftc.gov (search "consumer publications"). Be aware of substances that are banned by the military and various athletic associations.

## Table 14-1. Claims and Risks of Ergogenic Agents

| Type / Examples | Benefits / Risks / Side Effects |
|---|---|
| **Energy Enhancers**<br>Inosine, Coenzyme Q10 (COQ10), Desiccated Liver, Bee Pollen | No benefits demonstrated; some may increase free radical production or cause allergic reactions. |
| **Fat Burners / Lean Body Mass Enhancers**<br>L-Carnitine, Gamma Oryzanol, Ferulic Acid, Hydroxy-Methyl-Butyrate (HMB), Chromium Picolinate | No benefits demonstrated for many in this class. For HMB and chromium the research is inconclusive. Some may cause nausea, vomiting, cramps, and anemia. Chromium may cause DNA damage. |
| **Growth Hormone (GH) Releasers**<br>Arginine, Lysine, Ornithine, Branched chain Amino Acids (Leucine, Isoleucine, Valine), Free Amino Acids, Dibencozide, Cobamamide | Some benefits for Arginine, Lysine, and branched chain amino acids, but not the others. All may cause gastrointestinal (GI) upset, diarrhea, cramping, potential amino acid imbalances, and decreases in GH. |
| **CHO Sparers**<br>40-30-30, high fat/protein diets; Medium Chain Triglycerides (MCT); Ginseng; Lactate; Caffeine; Choline. | Some benefits reported for the diets; such diets may raise blood cholesterol and be a risk for heart disease. Some performance benefits for lactate and caffeine. No benefit demonstrated for others. Some may cause GI upset, allergic reactions, excitability, irritability, tremors, loss of concentration, nausea, and diarrhea. |
| **Testosterone Enhancers**<br>Glandulars (grounded organs); Sapogenins (Smilax, Diascorea, Trillium, Yucca, Sarsaparilla); Yohimbine; Boron; DHEA; Androstenedione, Andro, Androstenediol, Norandrostenediol; Steroids and steroid alternatives. | No benefits demonstrated; may cause testosterone production to decline and shrinking of the testicles; may cause light-headedness, aggression, nausea, vomiting, headaches, depression, lethargy, rashes, acne, and virilization in females. Some may increase risk of developing cancer. Andro group and other steroid alternatives are banned by the military. |
| **Intercellular Buffers**<br>Phosphate Salts; Aspartate Salts (Magnesium/ Potassium); Citrate; Sodium Bicarbonate. | Some benefits demonstrated for citrate and sodium bicarbonate, benefits are questionable for others. May cause GI upset, diarrhea, nausea, and cramps. |
| **Octacosanol (Wheat Germ Oil)** | Some benefits demonstrated in reaction times but not aerobic capacity; may cause allergic reactions. |
| **Glycerol** | No benefits demonstrated; may cause cellular dehydration, nausea, vomiting, and diarrhea. |

## Table 14-1. Claims and Risks of Ergogenic Agents

| Type / Examples | Benefits / Risks / Side Effects |
|---|---|
| **Omega-3 Fatty Acids** | No ergogenic effects have been demonstrated. |
| **Creatine** | Some performance benefits demonstrated during short-term, high intensity exercise, but benefits are negated if taken with caffeine. |
| **Tyrosine** | Some performance benefits demonstrated in mental tasks. |
| **Glutamine** | No performance benefits demonstrated. |
| **Glucosamine Sulfate with Chondroitin Sulphate** | Has potential for preventing and treating injuries, however is not endorsed by doctors due to the lack of research. |
| **Melatonin** | Benefits demonstrated; may cause sleepiness and fatigue at time of ingestion, but not upon awakening. |

# Ergolytic Agents

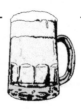

Ergolytic agents are those substances which impair physical and/or mental performance. When using these substances, you are undoing the benefits gained through training.

## Table 14-2. Ergolytic Agents and Performance

| Type / Examples | Side Effects / Risks |
| --- | --- |
| **Alcohol** | Heavy drinking can cause severe dehydration and decrease performance. |
| **Stimulants**<br>amphetamines, ephedrine | Banned by the military. These substances increase heart rate and blood pressure, can cause dizziness, stomach upset, irritability, insomnia, and death. |
| **Nicotine**<br>Cigarettes or Smokeless Tobacco | Increases heart rate and blood pressure, leading to decreased performance. |

# 15 | Training Issues for Women

In this chapter you will learn about:

- ♦ Guidelines for exercise during pregnancy and lactation.
- ♦ Female Athlete Triad.
- ♦ Eating Disorders.
- ♦ Osteoporosis.

Guidelines for nutrition and exercise for optimal health and performance are the same for women and men. However, special issues, such as pregnancy, will alter these practices. Seek the advice of your doctor.

## Pregnancy and Lactation

The American College of Obstetricians and Gynecologists (ACOG) has established guidelines for exercise during pregnancy. The general consensus is that women in good health may continue (or start) exercising during pregnancy. 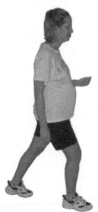 However, each woman should consult her doctor for personal recommendations as there are some contraindications to exercising during pregnancy. Proper nutrition and routine exercise during pregnancy is important for your health and the health of your baby. Table 15-1 outlines general nutrition and exercise guidelines that you should follow during pregnancy. The exercise guidelines have been adapted from ACOG's exercise guidelines.

**Table 15-1. Nutrition and Exercise Guidelines for Pregnant Women**

| Nutrition Guidelines | Exercise Guidelines |
|---|---|
| Choose nutrient dense foods (Chapter 3, page 20). | Exercise at least three times per week. Consult your doctor since there are some contraindications to exercising during pregnancy. |
| Eat according to the Food Guide Pyramid to meet your increased energy needs (Chapter 3). | Monitor exercise intensity according to perceived exertion or effort (Chapter 5). Target heart rate zone is not accurate since heart rate is higher during pregnancy. |
| Get adequate folate intakes prior to and during pregnancy to prevent birth defects (Chapter 2, Table 2-2). | Try swimming for low-impact aerobic exercise; water helps regulate body temperature. |
| Talk to your doctor about the proper amount of weight to gain for your pregnancy. | Stop exercise if you feel short of breath, feel any pain, feel dizzy or faint, or have contractions. |
| Meet nutritional demands for both pregnancy and exercise. You should not attempt to lose weight. | Avoid supine (lying on your back) exercises after the first three months of pregnancy. |
| Drink adequate amounts of water for both hydration and dissipation of heat. | Avoid activities that may result in trauma to the abdominal area, such as contact sports. |
| | Avoid exercises requiring balance, especially during the last three months of pregnancy. |
| | Avoid exhaustive and maximal exercise. |
| | Avoid exercising in environmental extremes. |
| | Avoid saunas, stream rooms, and whirlpools. |

# Nutrition and Exercise Guidelines for Lactating Women

After the baby's birth, gradually resume exercise, ultimately building up to your pre-pregnancy levels of duration and intensity. To lose weight after your pregnancy, do so according to the guidelines in Chapter 1 and the **Navy Nutrition and Weight Control Self-Study Guide** (NAVPERS 15602A). Consult your baby's pediatrician or your family physician with questions and concerns you have about your and your baby's diet. In general:

♦ Energy needs are higher when breast feeding than during pregnancy. Consume adequate kcals (roughly an extra 500 kcal per day).

♦ Choose nutrient dense foods (Chapter 3, page 20).

♦ Drink adequate fluids to prevent dehydration.

♦ Consume adequate calcium (see Chapter 2).

♦ Lactic acid production during exercise can affect the taste of breast milk, so breast feed prior to exercise.

- If you drink coffee, drink less than 2 cups a day; the caffeine may cause your baby to be sleepless and irritable.

- Avoid alcohol; alcohol enters the breast milk and can decrease the baby's appetite.

- Avoid cigarette smoking; smoking decreases milk production.

# Female Athlete Triad

The Female Athlete Triad is found among female athletes trying to balance the pressures of body image and physical performance. The triad (Figure 15-1), marked by inadequate food intake, menstrual abnormalities, and bone loss, can be fatal if left untreated. Therefore, a healthy relationship between food, body image, and performance must be established.

### Figure 15-1. The Female Athlete Triad

**Eating Disorders**
Dieting excessively to lose weight.
Compulsively overexercising.
Self-esteem governed by body weight.

Picture from FS Kaplan. Prevention and Management of Osteoporosis. CIBA Clinical Symposia. 47(1); 1995.

**Amenorrhea**
Irregular or absent menstrual cycles.

**Osteoporosis**
Weak bones.
Increased risk for fractures.

## Eating Disorders

An eating disorder results in inadequate intakes of kcals and nutrients to replenish the energy used during daily activities. Two common types of eating disorders are Anorexia Nervosa and Bulimia Nervosa. Some behaviors people with eating disorders engage in are starvation, self-induced vomiting, excessive exercise, and the misuse of laxatives or diuretics. Both disorders are extremely damaging to the mind and body, and, if untreated, can lead to death. These disorders can have long-term health consequences by affecting the heart, liver, kidneys, and bone. In addition, these behaviors severely limit physical and mental performance.

## Amenorrhea

A woman is considered amenorrheic when she misses three or more consecutive menstrual cycles. In well-nourished women, heavy physical training should not result in amenorrhea. When non-pregnant, premenopausal women become amenorrheic it may reflect malnutrition.

## Osteoporosis

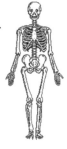

The decreased levels of female hormones during amenorrhea can lead to calcium loss from the bones and increase the likelihood of developing **osteoporosis** later in life. Osteoporosis is a major cause of bone fractures in the elderly. Bone density throughout the adult lifespan is greatly impacted by the amount of bone formed prior to the early thirties. Therefore, amenorrhea and eating disorders in young adults can negatively affect bone health for life. Prior to menopause, a healthy diet (including adequate calcium intakes) and the performance of weight bearing activities are the two factors that have the greatest positive influence on bone health (see Chapters 3, 4, 5, and 7).

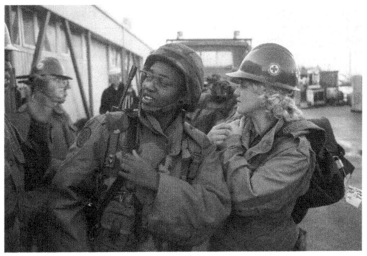

# 16 | Age and Performance

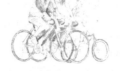

In this chapter you will learn about:

- ♦ Age-associated changes in metabolism and body composition.
- ♦ Countering age-associated changes in physical performance.

Aging is a natural process that most, if not all, people would like to avoid. Most people associate aging with gaining weight, getting weaker, and not being able to perform many of the activities they did in their youth. Many of these conditions are actually the result of inactivity, not aging. Although there are several inevitable physiologic changes that will occur as you age, the degree of these changes can be manipulated through sound dietary and exercise practices.

## Changes in Metabolism and Body Composition

Maintaining a healthy body weight and body fat percentage throughout your adult life is key to maintaining health and fitness as you age. This often seems easier said than done, considering basal metabolic rate (BMR, see Chapter 1) declines as you age.

>  With aging, expect to see a gradual decline in BMR, possibly resulting in needing 100 fewer kcal a day with each passing decade.
>
> Taken from Tufts University Health and Nutrition Letter. November 1998; 16(9): 6.

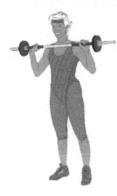

The loss of muscle mass as you age is directly responsible for the decline in BMR. Muscle is metabolically active, which means that it requires a set number of kcals each day to maintain its mass. On average, people begin to lose some muscle mass after the age of 35 years. This results in fewer metabolic demands and less total daily kcal requirements. However, the amount of muscle mass that you lose is dependent upon how much physical activity you perform as you age, particularly activities that require muscle strength such as strength training. By engaging in strength training exercises you will preserve and possibly gain muscle mass, leading to a 10% to 15% boost in your BMR!

Along with a decrease in muscle mass, inactivity can also lead to an increase in body fat. This occurs if the number of kcals consumed is greater than the number of kcals expended through physical activity, as explained in the energy balance equations in Chapter 1. This simultaneous increase in body fat and decrease in muscle mass leads to a greater body mass index (BMI) and is associated with an increased risk for heart and blood vessel diseases, obesity, diabetes, and other diseases (see Chapter 1).

Any alterations in energy expenditure, either through changes in BMR or changes in physical activity level, need to be countered by changes in kcal intake to keep your net energy balance at zero and to maintain your current body weight. Therefore, a combination of sound nutritional practices and regular physical activity will enable you to maintain a healthy body weight and body composition and remain physically fit as you age.

# Nutritional Needs

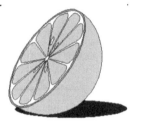

The Dietary Guidelines for Americans and the Food Guide Pyramid (outlined in Chapter 3) were designed to provide basic nutritional information and serve as educational tools for Americans over 2 years of age. Therefore, these guidelines should be followed to ensure good nutrition throughout your life. An important point to note is that although the age-related decline in BMR results in the need for fewer daily kcals, your requirements for nutrients such as vitamins, minerals, and proteins do not decrease with age (see Chapter 2). Therefore, proper food selection is essential to meet this challenge. Some ideas to help you meet your nutrient requirements without eating extra kcals include following the 5-A-Day campaign (eat at least five fruits and vegetables a day) and eating nutrient dense foods (see Chapter 3 and Appendix A).

# Countering Age-Associated Changes in Fitness

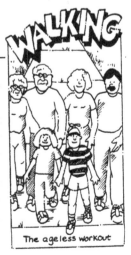

Ever heard the saying "use it or lose it?" This is true for physical fitness. Whether it is muscle strength or aerobic endurance, if you do not remain physically active as you age you cannot maintain the muscle mass or heart adaptations you need for peak performance (review the effects of detraining listed in Chapter 4). **Though effects of detraining listed in** Chapter 4). **Though** aging can lead to decreases in fitness levels, the amount of decline can be offset by a regular exercise routine. Therefore, age itself does not predispose you to have large decrements in physical performance.

The ageless workout

Some gradual changes you can expect in your physical performance as you age are listed below.

### Table 16-1. Age-Related Changes in Fitness

| Fitness Component | Typical Age-Related Change | Countermeasure |
|---|---|---|
| Aerobic Capacity | 5% to 15% decline each decade after the age of 30. | Do aerobic exercise regularly; try to maintain your exercise intensity (see Chapters 4,5,6). |
| Muscle Strength | Loss of muscle mass and strength. | Do strength exercises regularly; training effect is based on your exercise intensity (see Chapters 4,7,8,10, Appendix B) |
| Flexibility | Loss of range of motion at a joint or joints. | Do stretching exercises regularly to maintain joint range of motion and prevent injury. Warm-up before stretching (see Chapters 4,9). |
| Anaerobic Capacity | Greater decline than aerobic capacity. | Do speed work in addition to aerobic exercise only if you want to maintain performance-related fitness or participate in competitive sports (see Chapters 4,5). |

Other fitness issues to consider as you age include the following:

♦ **Warm-Up and Cool-Down** - Longer warm-up and cool-down times are needed to prepare your body for the upcoming exercise and reduce your risk of injury, particularly if you are participating in strenuous exercise (see Chapter 4).

♦ **Recovery from Workouts** - You will need to allow for longer recovery times from strenuous workouts and competition. You may actually notice this before you notice a decline in your performance. Allow for adequate recovery by following a hard workout with a couple rest days or light workout days. In addition, allow your body adequate time to adapt to increases in your workout. Pay attention to the warning signs of overtraining (see Chapter 13).

♦ **Recovery from Injuries** - As with recovery from a strenuous workout, you will probably need more time to recover from training injuries. Be patient and allow yourself to fully recover. This will help you avoid future injuries (see Chapter 13).

♦ **Cross-Training** -No specific exercise is better than another to offset all the health and fitness changes mentioned. However, many of these concerns can be addressed by cross-training, or altering the types of exercises you

106

perform, throughout the week (see Chapter 5). By cross-training, you can improve and maintain your aerobic fitness while recovering from intense workouts or while taking a break from weight-bearing exercises. This will help prevent overtraining and overuse injuries (see Chapter 13) while you remain physically active. So, consider making cross-training a regular practice in your exercise routine, if it is not already.

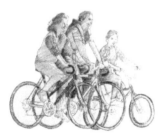

As you grow older your responsibilities, interests, leisure time activities, as well as your level of motivation may affect how physically active you are. However, it is important to remember that a sedentary or inactive lifestyle, combined with poor eating habits, can increase the risk for developing obesity, heart disease, strokes, diabetes, some types of cancers, high blood pressure and osteoporosis. Adopting sound eating and exercise habits (the earlier the better) can help reduce the risk for developing the above mentioned diseases. Chapter 17 provides information on how to develop and maintain healthy habits.

# 17 | Adopting Healthy Habits

In this chapter you will learn about:

- ◆ Setting SMART goals.
- ◆ Reaching goals.
- ◆ Evaluating progress.
- ◆ Staying motivated and overcoming setbacks.

Forming habits to enhance physical performance and for achieving a healthier lifestyle is both personally and professionally rewarding. Using the information provided in the preceding chapters, you can set goals, develop healthy habits and achieve your objectives. For example, if your objective is to improve cardiovascular fitness, use the information provided in Chapters 4, 5, 6, and 11 to design your a plan of action. Remember, effective programs for enhancing physical performance and overall health include both sound nutrition practices and appropriate physical training.

The process of developing and maintaining healthy habits can be challenging. It is a gradual process which requires commitment, effort and perseverance. Ultimately, the payoff will be in the form of enhanced job-related physical performance, being in great physical shape, and lowering your risk for developing chronic health problems as you get older. Everyone ages: steps you take now will last a lifetime!

## Setting "SMART" Goals

As you go through the process of changing and adopting healthy habits, you are actively taking charge of your health. Begin by setting Specific, Measurable, Action-oriented, Realistic and Timed (SMART) goals to meet your fitness and health-related objectives. A SMART goal should be:

- ◆ **Specific** - The more specific the goal, the easier it is to plan your routines to reach the goal. If you have a general goal, pick a specific area to focus on. For example, define "I want to increase my running distance" to "I will increase my running distance by one mile." Another example, restate "I want to increase my dietary fiber intake" as "I will add one additional serving each of fruits and vegetables to my daily diet".

- ◆ **Measurable** - Your specific goal should be easy for you to measure so you can chart your progress. Taking the running example above, you can easily measure the distance you run to determine if you are meeting your goal. As for the fiber example, you can record your fruit and vegetable intake (see Appendix A).

♦ **Action-oriented** - When defining a specific goal state exactly what actions you must do to achieve the goal. This becomes your plan to reach your goals. For example, "I will increase my run by a quarter mile every two weeks until I am able to run an additional mile."

♦ **Realistic** - Be realistic in your expectations of yourself and what you expect to gain. Taking large or long-term goals and breaking them into smaller, more manageable goals to keep you motivated and focused on your actions. For example, train for and run a 5k race, then build up to a 10k race.

♦ **Timed** - Time lines provide direction in planning short-term goals and actions to reach long-term goals and objectives. Using the running example above: two weeks is the deadline for increasing run distance by a quarter mile, and two months is the long-term deadline for increasing distance by one mile.

Table 17-1 lists a number of general nutrition and fitness-related goals to assist you in identifying your own goals and in designing and setting "SMART" goals as described above.

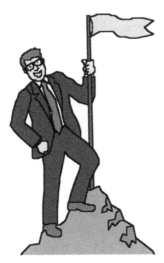

**Table 17-1. Some General Nutrition and Fitness-Related Goals**

| General Nutrition-Related Goals | General Fitness-Related Goals |
|---|---|
| ❏ Read food labels when buying foods. | ❏ Health benefits (lower cholesterol, lower blood pressure, and lower stress). |
| ❏ Eat foods according to their serving sizes. | ❏ Improve/maintain heart and lung (cardiovascular) fitness. |
| ❏ Eat at least 5 servings of fruits and vegetables each day. | ❏ Improve/maintain muscular strength. |
| ❏ Include foods that are good sources of calcium. | ❏ Improve performance of job-related physically-demanding tasks. |
| ❏ Follow the U.S. Dietary Guidelines. | ❏ Maintain healthy body weight and body fat. |
| ❏ Drink plenty of fluids to maintain fluid balance. | ❏ Improve/maintain flexibility. |
| ❏ Eat more dietary fiber. | ❏ Have strong bones. |
| ❏ Reduce saturated fat and cholesterol intakes. | ❏ Improve physical appearance. |
| ❏ Other:_____ | ❏ Other:_____ |

# Reaching Goals

The more specific and realistic your goals, the easier it will be to develop and follow action plans to meet these goals. More than likely, unforeseen events will lead to altered plans; expect this and keep your ultimate goals in mind when replanning. Next incorporate your plan into your daily routines. At first you will have to consciously make efforts to follow your plans, but, after continuous practice, these plans will become your new habit. The following points and the steps and actions listed in Table 17-2 will help you reach your goals:

♦ Start simple: pick a goal that you feel will be easy to achieve.

♦ Work toward one goal at a time.

♦ If you notice that you are having difficulty achieving a goal, revise your plan and alter your strategy.

**Table 17-2. Steps and Actions To Take To Reach Your SMART Goals**

| STEPS | ACTIONS |
|---|---|
| Develop | Develop an support system of friends, family and/or coworkers who will encourage you. |
| Make | Make change a priority; Make time; Remember you control your off-duty schedule. |
| Create | Create a plan of action -- one that works for you, motivates you and fits in your schedule. |
| Monitor | Monitor your progress -- use the tracking charts provided in Appendix A and Appendix B. |
| Reward | Reward yourself when you meet a goal. |
| Use | Use long-term vision. Remember healthy habits will greatly enhance the quality of your life in later years. |

Adapted from National Cancer Institute and Centers for Disease Control and Prevention (http://5aday. nci.nih.gov/).

# Maintaining Healthy Habits

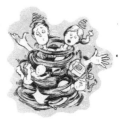

Once your "new" habit becomes a part of your routine and is performed effortlessly, you are maintaining, rather than adopting, this habit. Maintaining healthy habits during interruptions in your regular routine (such as vacations or illness) can create challenges of its own. So how can you maintain your routine when faced with setbacks?

♦ Anticipate and try to avoid setbacks or upsets to your routine.

♦ Plan in advance how you will handle interruptions (e.g.vacation) to your schedule.

♦ Motivate yourself to restart your routine when things "return to normal". For example, give your workout buddy $20 before you go on vacation to keep on your behalf until you restart your exercise routine.

♦ Reward yourself once you have achieved maintenance for your goal. The reward should be appropriate for the goal attained (preferably non-food). For example: put $1 in a piggy bank for every workout you complete for a month and use it to buy yourself new exercise gear or a ticket to your favorite sporting event.

♦ Enhanced fitness builds self-confidence which is a powerful motivator!

Ultimately, your perceptions of the health and fitness benefits associated with healthy eating practices and regular exercise are important for maintaining healthy lifestyle behaviors. We hope that the information provided in this guide motivates you to follow healthy nutrition and physical fitness practices.

# Appendix A: Ideas for Healthy Food Choices

Make gradual changes to your diet. Eating healthfully requires making overall smart food selections throughout your life. Choosing a food that is less nutritious every once in awhile does not mean your diet is bad; just make those foods the exception in your diet, not the rule.

**Table A-1. Healthier Food Selections**

| | Try: | In place of: |
|---|---|---|
| **Grains** | Whole grains and pastas, and brown rice. | Bleached, white, or processed varieties. |
| | Cooking pastas and rice in broths. | Cooking pastas and rice in water with butter. |
| **Vegetables/ Fruits** | Low-fat or non-fat salad dressings or vinagrette on salads. | Creamy salad dressings. |
| | Vegetables marinated in herbs and lemon or lime juice. | Adding butter to vegetables. |
| **Meats** | Canadian bacon or ham. | Bacon. |
| | Ground turkey, extra-lean ground beef, or lean, trimmed red meats. | Ground beef. |
| | 2 egg whites. | 1 whole egg. |
| | Poultry or fish. | Marbled red meats. |
| | Steaming, broiling, baking, or grilling. | Frying. |
| **Dairy** | Low-fat or non-fat sour cream, cottage cheese (whipped until smooth), or yogurt. | Sour cream. |
| | Skim milk. | Whole milk or nondairy creamer. |
| | Low-fat cheeses. | Cheese. |

## Table A-1. Healthier Food Selections

| | Try: | In place of: |
|---|---|---|
| **Fats** | Applesauce for baking. | Oil (1:1 substitution). |
| | Wine or broth-based sauces. | Cream and butter sauces. |
| | Canola, olive, and safflower oils. | Animal fats, coconut oil, and palm oil. |
| | Cocoa. | Chocolate. |
| | Spray butter or margarine. | Butter. |

## 5-A-Day Challenge

Some ideas to help you increase the number of fruits and vegetables you eat each day to meet the 5-A-Day challenge are: (see Table 3-1 for serving sizes.)

♦ Eat fruit or drink fruit juice at breakfast.

♦ Snack on fruits and vegetables (especially bite-sized portions such as baby carrots or dried fruits) throughout the day.

♦ Include one or more side servings of vegetables at lunch and dinner.

♦ Eat at least one **Vitamin A-rich fruit or vegetable** - good food sources include apricot, cantaloupe, carrot, mango, papaya, pumpkin, spinach, sweet potato, romaine lettuce, mustard greens, winter squash, kale, and collards.

♦ Eat at least one **Vitamin C-rich fruit and vegetable** - good food sources include orange, grapefruit, kiwi, apricot, pineapple, cantaloupe, strawberry, tomato, mango, plum, broccoli, cauliflower, brussel sprouts, peppers, collards.

♦ Eat at least one **Fiber-rich fruit and vegetable** - good food sources include apple, banana, berries, figs, prunes, cherry, kiwi, orange, date, pear, cooked beans (kidney, lima, pinto, black, lentils), black-eyed peas, peas, carrot, potato, and corn.

♦ Eat at least one **Cruciferous vegetable** (from cabbage family) - examples include broccoli, cauliflower, brussel sprouts, bok choy, red and green cabbage, kale, and turnip.

Remember: 5 fruits and vegetables a day is the minimum - more is better!

# Worksheet A-1. Nutrition Tracking Guide

| Food Groups | | Date: _____ | Date: _____ | Date: _____ | Date: _____ |
|---|---|---|---|---|---|
| | Grains & Cereals 6-11 servings | O O O O / O O O O / O O O | O O O O / O O O O / O O O | O O O O / O O O O / O O O | O O O O / O O O O / O O O |
| | Fruit 2-4 servings | O O O O | O O O O | O O O O | O O O O |
| | Vegetable 3-5 servings | O O O O O | O O O O O | O O O O O | O O O O O |
| | Meat & Meat Substitute 2-3 servings | O O O | O O O | O O O | O O O |
| | Dairy 2-3 servings | O O O | O O O | O O O | O O O |
| | Fats, Oils, & Sweets | Use Sparingly | Use Sparingly | Use Sparingly | Use Sparingly |

Note: See Chapter 3 for recommended number of servings and serving sizes. For a particular day, check off the number of servings you ate from each of the food groups. 1 circle - 1 serving.

115

# Appendix B: Sample Workout

This is a general cardiovascular and strength workout. Feel free to substitute or add exercises according to the guidelines described in Chapters 5 and 7. Use Worksheet B-1 and B-2 to design your workouts and chart your training progress. Seek help from the health promotion staff (CFC) if needed.

## Table B-1. Sample Workout

| Sequence | Activity | Frequency | Intensity | Time |
|---|---|---|---|---|
| **Warm-up** | | Before workout | 50% maxHR | 5 min. |
| **Aerobic** | Walk, Run, Swim, etc. | 3 to 7 days/week | 60 to 75% maxHR | 30 to 60 min. |
| **Cool-down** | | After workout | 100 bpm | 5 min. |
| **Strength** | | 3 days/week (Mon, Wed, Fri or Tues, Thurs, Sat) | 2 sets of 12 repetitions | 20 to 45min |
| Legs | Squats | | | |
| | Leg Curl | | | |
| Chest | Chest Press | | | |
| Back | Seated Row | | | |
| Shoulder | Lateral Raise | | | |
| Triceps | Triceps Extension | | | |
| Biceps | Biceps Curl | | | |
| Lower Back | Back Extension | | | |
| Abdominals | Ab Crunch | | | |
| | Side Crunch | | | |
| **Stretch** | | 3 to 7 days/week | 30 seconds X 2 | 10 min. |
| | Quadriceps | | | |
| | Hamstring | | | |
| | Pretzel | | | |
| | Butterfly | | | |
| | Chest | | | |
| | Upper Back | | | |
| | Rock-n-roll | | | |
| | Lizard | | | |

Note that the duration of this workout is dependent on the number of exercises that are performed and the length of the aerobic exercise. Perform the number and duration of exercises that are appropriate for your fitness level and adjust the routine as your fitness improves.

# Worksheet B-1. Aerobic Exercise Log

| Date: | | | | | | | |
|---|---|---|---|---|---|---|---|
| Type | | | | | | | |
| Heart Rate | | | | | | | |
| Time | | | | | | | |
| Comments | | | | | | | |
| Date | | | | | | | |
| Type | | | | | | | |
| Heart Rate | | | | | | | |
| Time | | | | | | | |
| Comments | | | | | | | |
| Date | | | | | | | |
| Type | | | | | | | |
| Heart Rate | | | | | | | |
| Time | | | | | | | |
| Comments | | | | | | | |
| Date | | | | | | | |
| Type | | | | | | | |
| Heart Rate | | | | | | | |
| Time | | | | | | | |
| Comments | | | | | | | |

Under "Type", list the workout you performed (i.e., running, walking). Under "Comments" note how you felt during exercise, your perceived exertion (6-20 on the Borg scale), or any other measure that you use to track your progress.

# Worksheet B-2. Strength Exercise Log

| Exercises: | Date:____ set x rep / wgt | Date:____ set x rep / wgt | Date:____ set x rep / wgt | Date:____ set x rep / wgt | Date:____ set x rep / wgt | Date:____ set x rep / wgt | Date:____ set x rep / wgt | Date:____ set x rep / wgt |
|---|---|---|---|---|---|---|---|---|
| **Chest** | / | / | / | / | / | / | / | / |
|  | / | / | / | / | / | / | / | / |
|  | / | / | / | / | / | / | / | / |
|  | / | / | / | / | / | / | / | / |
| **Back** | / | / | / | / | / | / | / | / |
|  | / | / | / | / | / | / | / | / |
|  | / | / | / | / | / | / | / | / |
|  | / | / | / | / | / | / | / | / |
| **Shoulders & Arms** | / | / | / | / | / | / | / | / |
|  | / | / | / | / | / | / | / | / |
|  | / | / | / | / | / | / | / | / |
|  | / | / | / | / | / | / | / | / |
| **Legs** | / | / | / | / | / | / | / | / |
|  | / | / | / | / | / | / | / | / |
|  | / | / | / | / | / | / | / | / |
|  | / | / | / | / | / | / | / | / |
| **Lower Back& Abs** | / | / | / | / | / | / | / | / |
|  | / | / | / | / | / | / | / | / |
|  | / | / | / | / | / | / | / | / |
|  | / | / | / | / | / | / | / | / |
| Remember to stretch! | | | | | | | | |

See Chapter 7 for strength training guidelines. Rep - repetition; Set - the number of reps performed without resting; wgt - weight lifted; Abs - abdominals

# Appendix C: Strength Exercises

**Legs**

### Squats
Place barbell across shoulders on upper back, not directly on neck. Keep head up, back straight, feet slightly wider than shoulder-width apart, and point toes out. Keep back perpendicular to deck. Count 1: Squat in a controlled motion until knees are over toes, but no lower than having your thighs parallel to deck. Inhale squatting down. Count 2: Return to start position, exhaling while standing up. Variation: 3/4 Squat - Squat until knees are at a 120° angle (half of the normal squat). Return to start position. Works quadriceps, hamstrings, gluteals, calves.

### Leg Press
Keep hips and back flat against support pad. Count 1: Slowly lower platform until knees are at a 90° angle. Inhale lowering platform. Count 2: Return to start position, exhaling while raising platform. Do not lock your knees. Works quadriceps and hamstrings.

### Standing Calf Raises
Place shoulders under pads of machine, balls of feet on foot rest. Count 1: Stand straight with knees slightly bent, rise up on toes as high as possible, keeping the balls of your feet in contact with the machine. Exhale lifting up. Count 2: Return to start position, inhaling while lowering weight. Do not lock knees. Works calves.

### Lunge
Stand with feet shoulder-width apart, bar resting on back of shoulders. Count 1: Take big step forward with one leg. Count 2: Squat straight down until the front leg's thigh is parallel to deck. Inhale when lunging. Do not let front knee bend so it moves in front of toes. Count 3: Stand up. Count 4: Push back to start position, exhaling when standing up. Repeat with other leg. Variation: Walking Lunge - perform lunges while alternating legs as you walk across the deck. Works hamstrings, quadriceps, gluteals, calves; can use dumbbells placed at your sides

### Leg Extensions
Sit on machine with feet under foot pad, lightly hold seat handles for support. Count 1: Keeping feet flexed, raise weight until legs are extended but knees are not locked. Exhale while extending legs. Do not bounce the weight. Count 2: Slowly return to start position, inhaling while lowering legs. Do not let weight drop. Works quadriceps.

### Seated Calf Raises
Place balls of feet on foot rest, pads resting on top of thighs. Count 1: Raise heels as high as possible. Exhale lifting up. Count 2: Slowly drop heels as low as possible. Inhale lowering weight. Works calves.

---

**Legs**

### Leg Curls
Place heels, with feet flexed, under foot pads so the pads are at the back of heels, not calves. Count 1: Curl legs up, bringing ankle pad close to your gluteals. Exhale curling legs up. Count 2: Return to start position, inhaling while extending legs. Do not lift hips or arch back during lift. Works hamstrings.

**Chest**

### Incline Dumbbell Press
Lie on 20° incline bench. Feet flat on deck. Hold the dumbells in front of shoulders, palms out. Count 1: Press dumbbells straight up until arms are extended. Exhale raising weight. Keep elbows slightly bent. Lower back should stay on the bench and back should be straight. Count 2: Return to start position, inhaling while lowering weight. Works chest, shoulders and arms.

### Cable Flys
Lie on bench with feet flat on deck. Grip cable handles with arms extended, palms up, and elbows slightly bent. Count 1: Bring arms up and over your chest, crossing them over your chest. Exhale while pulling cables across chest. Elbows should remain slightly flexed; but do not bend them more to pull the cables. Count 2: Return to start position, inhaling while extending arms. Keep upper arms in line with shoulders and collarbone during movement. Works chest.

### Dips
Rest hands on parallel bars. Extend arms; legs are not to support your weight unless needed for assistance. Count 1: Bend the elbows until shoulders are level with the elbows. Inhale while lowering body. Count 2: Extend arms to return to start position. Exhale while lifting body. Works triceps, chest and shoulders.

### Bench Press
Lie on bench with feet flat on deck. Hold barbell at arms length above mid chest with palms facing out. Count 1: Lower barbell until it barely touches your chest by bringing your elbows straight down and behind you. Inhale while lowering barbell. Do not bounce the bar off your chest. Count 2: Return to start position, exhaling while raising barbell. Variation: Use dumbbells. Works chest, shoulder and arms.

### Dumbbell Flys
Lie on bench with feet flat on deck. Hold dumbbells at arms length above upper chest with palms facing each other. Count 1: Keeping elbows slightly bent, lower dumbbells out to each side of chest in semi-circular motion. Dumbbells should be even with sides of chest. Inhale lowering dumbbells. Count 2: Return to start position, exhaling while raising dumbbells. Works chest.

### Curl Grip Pulldowns

Grab pulldown bar using underhand grip, arms extended shoulder-width apart. Sit on pad and keep back straight. Count 1: Pull bar down until it touches top of chest. Exhale on pull down. Do not swing or rock lower back during movement. Count 2: Return to start position, inhaling as you extend your arms. Works back and biceps.

### T-Bar Rows

Using a T-bar row machine, step onto foot supports and lie torso flat on support pad. Reach down and grab one set of handles on the T-bar with an overhand grip, hands shoulder width apart. Center and hold T-bar in extended arms. This is your start position. Count 1: Lift bar toward chest, pulling elbows straight up and behind you. Keep torso still on the support pad. Exhale when raising the T-bar. Count 2: Inhale while fully extending arms. Works back and arms.

### Seated Rows

Place feet against a stationary foot rest with knees slightly bent. Hold pulley bar at chest height with arms extended. Keep back straight. Count 1: Pull bar to middle of chest, keeping forearms parallel to deck. Exhale pulling arms back. Do not rock backwards or forward during movement. Count 2: Return to start position, inhaling while extending arms. Works back and arms.

### Lat Pulldowns

Grab pulldown bar using overhand grip, arms extended shoulder-width apart. Sit on pad and keep back straight. Count 1: Pull bar down by bringing elbows down to your sides until the bar touches your upper chest. Exhale on pull down. Do not arch your lower back during this exercise. Count 2: Return to start position, inhaling as arms extend. Works back and biceps.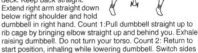

### One Arm Dumbbell Rows

Place left knee and hand on bench, extend right leg on deck. Keep back straight. Extend right arm straight down below right shoulder and hold dumbbell in right hand. Count 1:Pull dumbbell straight up to rib cage by bringing elbow straight up and behind you. Exhale raising dumbbell. Do not turn your torso. Count 2: Return to start position, inhaling while lowering dumbbell. Switch sides and repeat. Works back and biceps.

### Back Extensions

On a back extension bench, place your hip bones just over the front end of the front pad and your ankles under the rear pads. Count 1: Slowly bend at the waist, lowering your head to the deck. Bend at the waist and keep your back straight. Inhale when lowering torso. Count 2: Slowly lift your torso up until your back is parallel to the deck. Exhale when raising torso. Works lower back. For beginners, see the lower back exercises on pages 52 and 61.

---

### Rotating Dumbbell Curls

On incline bench, hold dumbbells with arms extended down, palms facing back. Count 1: As you begin to lift dumbbells, rotate hands so palms face up before they pass the bench pad. Keep palms up as you bring dumbbells up to shoulder. Exhale raising dumbbell. Count 2: Return to start position, rotating your palms to face back after they pass the bench pad. Inhale while lowering dumbbell. Works biceps.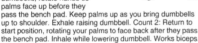

### Triceps Pressdown

Grab bar or rope with hands close together in center of body, elbows at $75^{\circ}$ so forearms are not quite parallel to deck. Push rope down until arms are straight, elbows remaining close to your sides. Exhale while pushing down. Count 2: Return to start position, inhaling while bringing forearms up. Works triceps.

### Wrist Curls

Grab a dumbbell or barbell palms up and sit on the edge of a bench. Place elbows on bench edge between knees. Let wrists hang over bench. Count 1: Curl wrists up to raise weight toward elbow. The motion should resemble a semi-circle. Exhale raising dumbbell. Keep forearms flat against bench through entire exercise. Count 2: Return to start position, inhaling while lowering weight. Works wrist flexors.

### Barbell Curls

Stand with feet shoulder width apart, back straight. Grab barbell with underhand grip, shoulder-width apart. Extend arms down, placing barbell against upper thighs. Count 1: Bend elbows and lift barbell toward chest. Keep elbows and arms close to sides. Do not throw weight up by arching back and swinging barbell. Do not rock elbows forward. Count 2: Return to start position. Exhale raising barbell, inhale lowering barbell. Works biceps.

### Tricep Extension with Barbell

Lie on bench with feet flat on deck, head at top of bench. Hold barbell above head with hands approximately 6"apart, palms up. Count 1: Lower bar to forehead, bending elbows. inhale lowering barbell. Upper arm should remain stationary. Count 2: Return to start position, exhaling while raising barbell. Works triceps.

### Reverse Wrist Curls

Grab a dumbbell or barbell palms down and sit on the edge of a bench. Place elbows on bench edge between knees. Let wrists hang over bench. Count 1: Curl wrists up to raise weight toward elbow. The motion should resemble a semi-circle. Exhale raising dumbbell. Keep forearms flat against bench through entire exercise. Count 2: Return to start position, inhaling while lowering weight. Works wrist extensors.

**Upright Rows**

Hold barbell with narrow overhand grip. An E-Z curl bar is suggested. Hands should be no more than 6 inches apart. Stand straight, hold barbell against upper thighs at arms length. Count 1: Keeping bar close to body and back straight, pull bar upward until just under chin. Arms should form a slight "v" at top of movement. Exhale raising bar. Keep elbows out and up. Count 2: Return to start position, inhaling while lowering bar. Works shoulders.

**Shoulder Press**

Sit with back straight and against support pad; keep feet flat on the deck. Incline bench 5-10˚, if possible. Raise dumbbells to shoulder height, palms facing forward. Keep elbows out. Count 1: Raise dumbbell overhead until arms are extended, slight bend in elbow. Count 2: Return to start position. Exhale raising weights, inhale lowering weights. Works shoulders.

**Internal Rotators**

Hold a dumbbell in left hand and lie on a bench on your left side. Bend left elbow 90°. Count 1: Rotate left upper arm so left hand is lifted up toward your right side. Exhale on lift. Do not move torso during exercise. Count 2: Return to start position, inhaling while lowering your left forearm. Works internal shoulder rotators. Switch sides to work right shoulder.

**External Rotators**

Hold a dumbbell in right hand and lie on a bench on your left side. Bend right elbow 90°. Count 1: Rotate right upper arm so right hand moves down toward left side. Inhale while lowering right forearm. Do not move torso during exercise. Count 2: Rotate right upper arm so right hand moves up above your right side. Exhale when lifting weight. Works internal shoulder rotators. Switch sides to work right shoulder.

General training mistakes that you should be aware of and avoid include:

♦ Locking joints at the end of their range of motion. This places a lot of stress on the joint. You should extend the joint as far as possible without locking it during your exercises.

♦ Moving your legs or "bouncing" during exercises. If you have to move or bounce body parts that are not directly involved in the exercise to lift a weight, then the weight is too heavy. Lower the weight and check your form by focusing on how your body is moving; do not focus on lifting the weight.

♦ Lifting and lowering weights rapidly. This can lead to injury. Slowly return the weight to the starting position, as this is the part of the workout that results in the greatest training effects!

# Appendix D: Resources

♦ This manual can be found on the internet at both the Uniformed Services University of the Health Sciences (under Academics, Military and Emergency Medicine, Human Performance Lab) and the Navy Environmental Health Center (NEHC) Health Promotion web sites (addresses listed on page 111). In addition, other health promotion materials for Navy personnel can be found on NEHC's web site.

♦ E. Aaberg. *Resistance Training Instruction*. Champaign, IL: Human Kinetics, 1999.

♦ American College of Obstetricians and Gynecologists. Women's Health Pamphlets. Washington, DC. 1994. (202-863-2518.)

♦ American College of Sports Medicine. Exercise and Physical Activity for Older Adults. 1998 Position Stand. *Medicine and Science in Sports and Exercise* 1998;30(6):992-1008.

♦ TR. Baechle (Ed.) *Essentials of Strength Training and Conditioning*. Champaign, IL: Human Kinetics, 1994.

♦ RC Cantu and LJ Micheli (Eds.). *ACSM's Guidelines for the Team Physician*. Philadelphia: Lea & Febiger, 1991.

♦ M. Cibrario. *A Complete Guide to Rubberized Resistance Exercises*. Mundelein, IL: Spri Products, Inc.

♦ Committee on Dietary Allowances. Recommended Dietary Allowances, 10th ed. Washington, DC: National Academy Press, 1989.

♦ R. Cotton (Ed.) (1996) *Lifestyle and Weight Management Consultant Manual*. San Diego, CA; American Council on Exercise.

♦ LT L. Cox. (1996) *Navy Nutrition and Weight Control Self-Study Guide*. NAVPERS 15602A. (http://www.bupers.navy.mil; click "Services"; click "Navy Nutrition and Weight Control.")

♦ L. Cox. Seaworthy. *Women's Sports and Fitness* July-August 1995;17(5):73-75.

♦ Defense Visual Imaging Center. http://www.dodmedia.osd.mil/. Navy photos.

♦ PA. Deuster, A. Singh, and P. Pelletier. *The Navy SEAL Nutrition Guide*. Washington D.C.; Government Printing Office. 1994.

♦ PA. Deuster (Ed.) *The Navy SEAL Physical Fitness Guide*. Washington D.C.; Government Printing Office. 1997

♦ JL. Durstine, et. al. (Eds) *ACSM's Resource Manual for Guidelines for Exercise Testing and Prescription. 2nd ed*. Baltimore: Lea & Febiger. 1993.

♦ J. Ellis with J. Henderson, *Running Injury-Free*, Rodale Press, 1994.

♦ W. Gain and J. Hartmann. *Strong Together! Developing Strength with a Partner.* Toronto: Sports Books Publisher, 1990.

♦ E. Howley and BD. Franks, Health *and Fitness Instructor's Handbook, 2nd ed.* Champaign, IL: Human Kinetics, 1992.

♦ Institute of Medicine. *Assessing Military Readiness in Women: The Relationship Between Body Composition, Nutrition, and Health.* Washington, D.C.: National Academy Press, 1998.

♦ DT. Kirkenall and WE. Garrett, Jr. The Effects of Aging and Training on Skeletal Muscle. *American Journal of Sports Medicine* 1998; 26(4):598-602.

♦ F. Koch. *Strength Training for Sports*; Applied Futuristics$^{SM}$, 1994.

♦ SJ. Montain, WA. Latzka, and MN Sawka. Fluid Replacement Recommendations for Training in Hot Weather. *Military Medicine* 1999;164(7):502-508.

♦ OPNAVINST 6110.1E. March 23, 1998. (http://neds.nebt.daps.mil/ directives/6110_1e.pdf)

♦ B. Pearl and G. Morgan. *Getting Stronger.* Bolinas, CA: Shelter Publications Inc. 1986.

♦ B. Rodgers and S.Douglas. Adjusting to Aging. American Running & Fitness Association, 1998. http://www.arfa.org.

♦ RJ. Shephard. Aging and Exercise. In: *Encyclopedia of Sports Medicine and Science*, TD. Fahey (Ed.) Internet Society for Sport Science: **Error! Hyperlink reference not valid.**. March 7, 1998.

♦ M. Sudy (Ed.). *Personal Trainer Manual: The Resource for Fitness Instructors.* Boston: Reebok University Press, 1993.

♦ *Tufts University Health & Nutrition Letter.* Outpacing Middle-Age Spread: Running. November 1998, page 6.

♦ EN. Whitney, CB. Cataldo, and SR. Rolfes. Understanding *Normal and Clinical Nutrition*, 5th ed. Wadsworth Publishing Company, 1998.

♦ US Dept. of Agriculture and US Dept. of Health & Human Services. *Nutrition and Your Health: Dietary Guidelines for Americans*, 4th ed. 1995.

♦ Peak Performance

# World Wide Web Sites (http://...)

| | |
|---|---|
| US Navy (Link to Navy Commands) | www.navy.mil (www.navy.mil/nol) |
| Uniformed Services University of the Health Sciences (USUHS), Human Performance Laboratory | www.usuhs.mil/acad/ index.html (select "Human Performance Laboratory" under Military and Emergency Medicine" |
| Navy Bureau of Personnel PRT standards Navy Nutrition and Weight Control Self-Study Guide | www.bupers.navy.mil/ services/ under "new PRT" /services under "Navy Nutrition..." |
| Navy Environmental Health Center Health Promotions-(NEHC) Fitness Site Nutrition Site | www-nehc.med.navy.mil/ hp/index.htm -.../hp/fitness/ index.htm.../hp/nutrit/index. htm |
| Naval Health Research Center (NHRC) | www.nhrc.navy.mil |
| American Alliance on Health, Physical Education, Recreation, and Dance (AAHPERD) | www.aahperd.org |
| American College of Sports Medicine (ACSM) | www.acsm.org |
| American Council on Exercise (ACE) | www.acefitness.org |
| American Dietetic Association | www.eatright.org |

| | |
|---|---|
| American Heart Association (AHA) | www.aha.org |
| American Running and Fitness Association (AR&FA) | americanrunning.org |
| Centers for Disease Control (US surgeon general's report) | www.cdc.gov (/nccdphp/ sgr/summ.htm) |
| National Academy of the Sciences Dietary Reference Intakes (DRIs) | www.nas.edu/ 276a.html and 287e.html |
| National Coalition to Promote Physical Activity (NCPPA) | www.ncppa.org |
| National "5-A-Day" campaign websites | 5aday.nci.nih.gov www.5ADAY.com |
| National Institutes of Health (NIH) Office of Dietary Supplements (ODS) | odp.od.nih.gov/ods/default. html |
| National Strength and Conditioning Association | www.nsca-lift.org |
| SCAN's Sports, Cardiovascular and Wellness Nutritionists | www.Nutrifit.org |
| US Department of Agriculture (USDA) | www.usda.gov |
| Shape Up America! | www.shapeup.org |

| US Food and Drug Association (FDA) | www.fda.gov |
| US Federal Trade Commission | www.ftc.gov |
| US Dept. of Health and Human Services | www.dhhs.gov |

Note: Addresses for web sites may change. If you are not able to access a site, try to contact the parent organization or search for their new site using a web browser.

# Glossary

acclimation - adaptations that occur within the body when exposed to a new environment.

aerobic capacity - maximal amount of aerobic activity that can be done

aerobic energy system - process of making energy (ATP) that requires oxygen.

amenorrhea - the cessation of menstruation not due to pregnancy or menopause; can be seen in women athletes whose nutritional intake is not adequate; one component of the female athlete triad.

anaerobic energy system - process of making energy (ATP) without using oxygen.

antioxidants - compounds that prevent breakdown (oxidation) of substances in the body; nutrients such as Vitamin E and C have antioxidant properties.

basal metabolic rate - the amount of energy (kcals) required to maintain life when the body at rest (BMR).

body composition - a description of the amount of body weight that is lean body mass (muscle, bones) and the amount of body weight that is fat.

body mass index (BMI) - an index that looks at weight in relation to height.

Calorie - a measure of energy used to describe the energy consumed in foods and expended through physical activity; Calorie with a capital "C" is the same as kilocalorie (kcal).

carbohydrates (CHO) - a macronutrient that supplies 4 kcals per gram; primary nutrient found in the grain, vegetable, and fruit food groups of the Food Guide Pyramid.

carbohydrate loading- nutritional training method used by endurance athletes to increase the amount of glycogen stores in their muscles before a competition.

cardiorespiratory fitness - ability of the heart, lungs, and blood vessels to deliver oxygen-rich blood to and remove waste products from the exercising muscles; the more trained the person, the higher the cardiorespiratory capacity; see aerobic capacity.

cholesterol - a substance made by the body that serves as a base for hormones such as estrogen and testosterone, is a part of all cells, and is consumed in the diet by eating animal products.

dehydration - a depletion of bodily fluids that occurs when not enough fluids are drunk to replace those lost through breathing, urination, and sweating.

detraining - a loss of training adaptations that occurs when training stops; can be avoided, stopped or reversed through physical training.

electrolytes - minerals in the body that help regulate fluid balance, are part of nerve conduction, and other essential bodily functions; examples include sodium, potassium, and chloride.

energy balance - net metabolism balance of the total kcals eaten minus the total kcals expended through basal metabolism and physical activity.

ergogenic agent - nutritional supplement taken with the purpose to enhance physical performance; examples include creatine, ginseng, caffeine and DHEA. many claim to improve performance but few have been demonstrated to be beneficial; may have health risks associated with long-term use.

ergolytic agent - supplement taken with the purpose to enhance physical performance but actually decreases performance; many have health risks associated with long-term use; examples include alcohol and nicotine.

| | |
|---|---|
| fat - | a macronutrient that supplies 9 kcals per gram; primary nutrient found in oils and butter; placed at the top of the Food Guide Pyramid. |
| female athlete triad - | cessation of menstrual cycles, loss of bone, and eating disorders seen in some women who participate in strenuous physical activity. |
| FITT Principle - | combination of four training factors (frequency, intensity, time, and type) that determine how an individual adapts to physical training. |
| flexibility - | the range of motion around a joint. |
| fluid balance - | net amount of fluid consumed minus the fluid lost through breathing, urine, and sweat. |
| glucose - | a simple CHO that serves as the main fuel to make energy (ATP) in the body. |
| glycogen - | a storage form of glucose found in muscles and liver. |
| heart rate (HR) - | the number of heart beats per minute. |
| kilocalorie (kcal) - | a measure of energy used to describe the energy consumed in foods and expended through physical activity. |
| kilogram (kg) - | metric measurement for weight; 1 kg = 2.2 pound (lbs). |
| lactic acid (lactate) - | a by-product of the anaerobic energy system. |
| ligament - | connective tissue that holds one bone to another bone. |
| macronutrient - | a nutrient that supplies kcals for energy metabolism; the three macronutrients are carbohydrate, protein, and fat. |
| metabolism - | chemical and physical processes that are required to maintain life. |
| METs - | metabolic equivalents; arbitrary unit of work in relation to rest; e.g., rest is 1MET, so if you exercise at 5METs you are expending 5 times the kcals you do at rest. |

| | |
|---|---|
| micronutrients - | nutrients that are needed in small amounts to aid in metabolism and other important bodily functions. micronutrients do not supply any kcals; the two classes are vitamins and minerals. |
| minerals - | class of micronutrient; examples of minerals are calcium, sodium, and potassium. |
| muscle endurance - | the ability of a muscle or muscle group to generate a less than maximal force over a period of time. |
| muscle strength - | the maximum force generated by a muscle or muscle group. |
| nutritional supplement- | a substance taken in addition to eating food to increase the amount of a particular nutrient or group of nutrients in the body. Some substances may also be taken in an attempt to improve physical performance. |
| osteoporosis - | a common bone disorder that is characterized by low bone density and weakened bones; people with osteoporosis have a greater risk of fracturing bones. |
| overhydration - | a gain of body water that occurs when too much plain water is drunk in an attempt to replace the fluid and electrolytes lost through sweating during strenuous and prolonged exercise; can be avoided by drinking a carbohydrate-electrolyte drink, such as a sports beverage, or eating a snack when exercising for more than 60 minutes. |
| overload - | placing greater-than-normal physical demands on the body with the intent of improving physical fitness and capability; this overload should be progressively increased. |
| overtraining syndrome - | a set of symptoms that are experienced when too much or too intense a physical activity is performed without adequate rest. |

oxygen consumption -     measure of the intensity of a physical activity. Maximal oxygen consumption ($VO_{2max}$) is a measure of the maximum work that an individual can perform both aerobically and anaerobically.

physical activity -     movement of the muscles that results in energy expenditure.

physical fitness -     the ability to perform physical activity.

pounds (lbs) -     measure for weight; 2.2 lbs = 1 kilograms (kg).

protein -     a macronutrient that supplies 4 kcals per gram; primary nutrient found in the dairy and meat / meat substitute food groups of the Food Guide Pyramid.

repetition -     one lifting and lowering of a weight or resistance during muscle training; often abbreviated "rep."

set -     a series of repetitions performed one after another without a rest period.

SMART goals -     defined goals that are specific, measurable, action-oriented, realistic, and timed.

specificity of training -     a principle which describes that training adaptations are optimized in a specific physical activity when that activity is performed in training sessions.

target heart rate zone-     a recommended heart rate range specific to each person, dependent on age and fitness level, that is within a safe intensity level to exercise.

tendon -     connective tissue that holds a muscle to a bone.

Valsalva maneuver -     when an individual holds his breath and bears down. This is impedes blood flow, increases blood pressure, and can be dangerous.

vitamins -     class of micronutrient; can be fat or water soluble; do not provide energy but are needed in many important functions; excessive intakes can be toxic.

waist-hip-ratio (WHR)-   a ratio of the waist circumferences (in inches) to the hip circumference (in inches); used to describe the distribution of body fat.

WATT -   measurement of work that describes the amount of kcals expended in a given time period; i.e., kcals/min.

Made in United States
Orlando, FL
29 November 2022

25216208R00076